FROM THE RIVER OF HEAVEN

Hindu and Vedic Knowledge
for the Modern Age

Other Passage Press Books by David Frawley

THE ASTROLOGY OF THE SEERS
A Guide to Vedic (Hindu) Astrology

AYURVEDIC HEALING
A Comprehensive Guide

BEYOND THE MIND
(Forthcoming)

GODS, SAGES AND KINGS
Vedic Secrets of Ancient Civilization

THE SONG OF THE SUN
The Upanishadic Vision
(Forthcoming)

WISDOM OF THE ANCIENT SEERS
Secrets of the *Rig Veda*
(Forthcoming)

FROM THE RIVER OF HEAVEN

Hindu And Vedic Knowledge for the Modern Age

by David Frawley

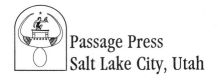

Passage Press
Salt Lake City, Utah

Passage Press is a division of Morson Publishing
Morson Publishing
P.O. Box 21713
Salt Lake City, Utah 84121-0713

All translations from the Sanskrit by David Frawley

Printed on acid-free paper

ISBN 1-878423-01-0

CONTENTS

Contents

Contents 7

Summary of the Source Teachings; Sacred History and Cosmology

Contents 7

Summary of the Source Teachings; Sacred History and Cosmology

Appendices 153

Contents   7

Summary of the Source Teachings; Sacred History and Cosmology

Contents

Contents 7

Summary of the Source Teachings; Sacred History and Cosmology

Contents 7

Summary of the Source Teachings; Sacred History and Cosmology

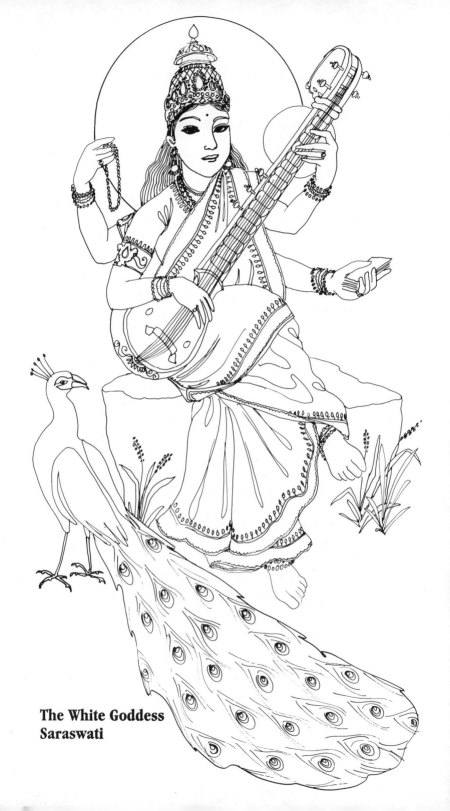

**The White Goddess
Saraswati**

True knowledge comes from the inside, not from the outside. It proceeds through the power of the Divine Word in the heart, not by the cunning of the human mind. It is the grace of the White Goddess, the Goddess of Wisdom, the great muse of the soul, who has many forms in all the lands and literatures of the world.

In the Hindu and Vedic tradition she is called Saraswati, She of the flowing stream of inspiration. She is the great stream of consciousness on whose banks the wise perform their rituals and their meditations. She is the great mother of the Vedas, the ancient books of wisdom.

She carries in her hands a rosary, a book, and plays the Vina. Her vehicle is the peacock, whose tail shows the manifold colors of her creative force. Her mantra is AIM.

She is the river of heaven, the milky way, the cosmic mother, by whose stream we speak, create and understand. This book is dedicated to her, as it proceeds by her power and her name.

> *Whose infinite, unencompassed, brilliant, moving flood, impetuously continues to roar, Who has filled the earthly regions and the wide realm of the atmosphere, may Saraswati protect us from blame.*
>
> *May the Goddess Saraswati, with all power, full of power, further us, as the guide of our minds.*
>
> *— Bharadwaja, Rig Veda VI. 61. 9, 11, 3*

PREFACE

The following book covers a large area of thought and experience in the oldest and most comprehensive spiritual tradition in the world. As such it is only meant to provide an overview and a glimpse of the many facets of this vast teaching. In many ways, therefore, it must be deficient. All the great teachers and teachings in the tradition could not be mentioned. Should some be left out, it does not mean that they are less important or significant than those included.

Nor do we have the space to provide references to follow up on all the ideas given in the different chapters. Many of the source teachings indicated have a number of translations available, which can be examined. Hence, the implementation of this book is your responsibility as the reader. You should begin to explore the teachings in your own right, seeking them not only outwardly but within your own heart. Should you make this effort the light and the grace to follow them must come to you.

FROM THE RIVER OF HEAVEN is part of a series of books which address many of these different facets of the Hindu and Vedic spiritual tradition. Such additional books can be examined for more detail on these subjects. We also welcome anyone who wishes to contribute to this approach. May the eternal and universal teaching (Sanatana Dharma) arise again!

✱✱✱

Of the teachers and teachings in my own experience, I would like to acknowledge Ramana Maharshi, the great guru of the path of knowledge; Sri Anandamayi Ma, who opened the light of devotion for me; the teachers of the Kriya Yoga lineage, for providing the great techniques of yoga; Sri Aurobindo and his disciples, for opening up the Vedic vision; Swami Rama Tirtha, for the gift of his ecstasy; and Swami Vivekananda, for beginning this great dissemination of the dharma to the West.

There is only one true religion, the religion of Truth.
There is only one true savior, the Divine Self within our Hearts.
There is only one true scripture, the Divine Word of Oneness.
Namaste!
Reverence to the Divine Spirit within you.

David Frawley
Santa Fe, New Mexico
February 1990

1
HINDU AND VEDIC KNOWLEDGE
IN THE MODERN AGE

Over the past century various spiritual teachers have come to the western world from India. Many of the teachings of the Indian spiritual tradition have also become available. They have made their imprint on our culture and on our language. This influence is one of the main factors, if not the most important, in the New Age culture emerging today and has become one of the primary forces of conscious change in the world. Such terms as guru and avatar, ideas as karma and reincarnation, Self-realization and God-realization, such practices as Yoga, meditation, vegetarianism and non-violence, all arise from the spiritual matrix of India. While the eastern world is under the influence of western culture on a technological and scientific level, the West in return is experiencing the spiritual side of culture preserved better in the East, particularly in India, the ancient land of religion.

Emerson and Thoreau, America's own great early teachers, first brought attention to the teachings of India in the middle of the nineteenth century. H.P. Blavatsky and the Theosophical Movement followed in the later part of the century; many of their teachings were based on Hindu and Buddhist sources from the great masters of the Himalayas. The first important teacher to arrive in this country from India was young Swami Vivekananda in the eighteen nineties, bringing over the teachings of his great master, regarded by many as an avatar or incarnation of God, Ramakrishna. A few years later came Swami Rama Tirtha for a brief but inspiring stay. In 1920 Paramahansa Yogananda became the first great teacher from India to establish his residency here. Since then many other yogis, swamis and gurus have come, or have sent their representatives or teachings. Today an ever increasing number visit, work or reside here. It would require a catalog to list them all.

Most known of these teachings is the practice of Yoga itself. The teachers of India chose the term Yoga from the many names of their tradition in order to appeal to the Western mind which is in revolt from dogmatic religious beliefs. Yoga is a neutral term for the practices, free of any cultural or intellectual bias. Of Yoga it is the physical side of Yoga, called Hatha Yoga, the science of postures, that we are most familiar with.

Yet this is only one aspect, the most visible rung of a great system of knowledge which includes all aspects of life and links all of life with the evolution of consciousness.

Previous to the journeys of these great teachers Vedic and Yogic knowledge was largely kept in secret in India, preserved mainly for the worthy or select few. For these modern teachers to make the trip to the West was a break from tradition. It is not that the Yogic teaching was always kept hidden. Previous teachers from India, not only Buddhists, but also Hindus, travelled to Rome in the West, to Indonesia and China in the East. Hinduism itself prevailed as far east as Indonesia until the sixteenth century.

The Yogic teaching was made secret largely as a defensive measure from repeated foreign invasions, mainly from the west of India. The Persians, Greeks, Huns, Scythes, Muslims and finally the British and Portuguese made India their target. Invasion followed invasion for over two thousand years. And whenever a culture is attacked it tends to become contracted. Hence, the closed nature the teaching assumed in the Middle Ages is not characteristic of its true nature which is open to all humanity but does not seek to impose itself on anyone. Its original openness has manifested again by the great world dissemination of Yoga that we see today.

VEDA AND YOGA

All knowledge has two sides; theory and practice. In the spiritual systems of India, Vedic science presents the theory and the systems of Yoga are the practice. They are the spiritual side of the religion we know as Hinduism. Veda itself means knowledge, wisdom or vision (as in our related European words of wit and wisdom from the German, idea, originally widea, from the Greek and video from the Latin). Yoga itself means the practical application of knowledge. It is harnessing the energy developed through knowledge to achieve the maximum integration of our being.

Hence, Veda and Yoga are one as theory and practise. Those who try to divide them up do not understand them. Both are aspects of an ancient universal spiritual science which we are again today seeking to restore as part of our movement towards a global culture.

THE RELEVANCE OF VEDIC SCIENCE

Vedic science is a system of spiritual knowledge encompassing all domains of life. First, it gives us the knowledge whereby liberation or self-realization can be gained, whereby we gain the true goal of life which is the immortality of our inner consciousness. Second, it provides the knowledge whereby the outer aspects of our lives can be harmonized with our spiritual purpose. This includes how to take care of our physical body and our society. As such Vedic knowledge provides the foundation for a true and spiritual human culture. It extends into all spheres of life and knowledge including medicine, astrology, mathematics, psychology, sociology and linguistics. It is the basis of the art of India, its poetry, music, dance and sculpture. It was the model for the social structure and legal system of ancient India, which was quite different in the Vedic age than in medieval or modern times.

Modern science is now entering into the subtle realms of mind and nature. It is beginning to see the inner side of the world and thus coming closer to the views of the ancient mystics. Such concepts as the relativity of time and space, are well known in Vedic science. To the ancient seers the entire universe is the creation (or recreation) of consciousness itself, with time and space as constructs of the mind. As such, they never looked upon time and space as having an ultimate or objective reality.

The Gaia hypothesis much talked about today in scientific circles, that there is a guiding life and intelligence on Earth, is another old Vedic idea. Gaia is Greek for Vedic Gau, the cosmic cow, the spirit or Goddess of the Earth, the Divine power working through it. The ancients had many chants to this Earth Goddess to insure the harmony of man and nature and to keep us attuned to the cosmic creative vibration. Some gave reverence to her, others sought to bring the Divine light, the power of the Gods into her. Such chants (like the Gayatri) give life to Gaia and protect and nourish all life on earth. Vedic science sees the universe as a magical play in the mind, a manifestation of cosmic law to demonstrate the glory of consciousness and the wonder of being.

As our materialistic science breaks through the ideas of time and space, we must begin to see the value of a spiritual science, a science of consciousness which encompasses all of life, outer and inner, a science of the eternal and the infinite. To rebuild such a spiritual science, we can find much of value in the ancient Vedic and Hindu teachings. This does not mean that we need only follow what remnants of Vedic science we have left today. Nor does it mean that India today is a model culture for the world to follow. Much of the ancient system is fragmented, scattered and worn by time. We need to recreate it and integrate it into our own lives and our own world situation. It is not a new science for us to become slaves of but a way of knowledge that gives freedom, which awakens creative intelligence and allows us to go beyond all dependency upon external forms. A science which rules us is a form of ignorance (nescience). It is the test of true knowledge that it gives freedom to both the mind and heart and helps us to understand and respect all humanity and all of life.

EAST AND WEST

Many of us in the western world tend to reject anything that originates in the East, because we see it as the imposition of a foreign and inappropriate culture upon us. We don't like to see such important cultural values as our religion, our language or way of life altered. We should note that people in the eastern world are struggling with the influence of western culture which they similarly feel is threatening to their cultural values. All human beings like to preserve their own culture and find other cultures hard to understand. In our examination of other cultures it is always easier to see their negative side. On the other hand, we are all exporting our cultures. Much more of the influence of western culture is still going to the East than that of the East is coming to the West. Yet neither culture can expect it to go only one way.

We are living at a time in which the influence of the East is starting to come to the West. In the previous centuries it has largely been the influence of the West going to the East with conquest and colonization followed by the export of western culture and religion and the technological and scientific knowledge developed in the West.

We must all realize, therefore, that the boundaries between East and West have been obliterated by modern communication. We cannot isolate ourselves from eastern cultural influences any more than they can isolate themselves from ours. Whereas western culture provides the world many gifts of science, technology and humanism, eastern culture provides those of spirituality and religion. Just as science and technology can be abused and cause much damage to the world, as we are witnessing today with pollution and the destruction of the environment, so too, eastern spiritual knowledge has its negative side, with some of the false guru cults and the corruption around them which are also visible today. Just as we need not reject science because of its misapplication, so too we should not reject the spiritual sciences of the East because of their misapplication.

Just as people of the eastern world can become adept at science and technology and can add many new insights and discoveries to it, so can many of us in the western world gain spiritual knowledge and become capable of adapting or developing it further. As we are now open to all the knowledge of the world, it no longer matters so much where we are born. We are less tied to our local culture and better able to perceive things for their own worth. We do not reject a peach because it is originally a fruit from China. So too, knowledge has an intrinsic value apart from its cultural context and this we should be open to that we might fully benefit from our complete human heritage.

Such divisions as East and West are simplistic ideas. They exaggerate geographical or cultural differences. We label the greater part of the world to be the East. Everything east of Europe is seen as the East, even though such cultures as India and China are quite distinct. They are as different from each other as our culture is from theirs. In many respects the culture of India stands in the center between the eastern influences of China and the western influences of Europe. For example, Hinduism contains the same religious teachings of devotion to God, as does the Judaeo-Christian-Islamic tradition to the west, as well as the formless meditative approaches of Buddhism and Taoism which prevail to the east. As such it affords a good point of integration for East and West.

VEDIC KNOWLEDGE IN WESTERN CULTURE

All culture is composite in nature, and different aspects of our culture come from different sources. Our religions, Christianity and Judaism, come from an ancient Middle Eastern cultural matrix. Most of the secular part of our culture, science, art, and philosophy comes from a Greco-Roman base. Our languages and our folk culture derives mainly from our Germanic, Slavic or Keltic ancestors. There is even an Indian or Vedic influence in our culture.

The further we trace back Indo-european languages the more they come to resemble Sanskrit. These include the Germanic, Slavic, Keltic, Greek and Latin tongues of most of Europe. Ancient Sanskrit has many words we would find familiar: matar, mother; pitar, father; duhitar, daughter; sunu, son; svasar, sister; bhratar, brother; gau, cow. Such words generally relate to the most fundamental factors of life.

In terms of language, western or European culture has a common root with the Sanskrit. In terms of culture, many of the practices of ancient European religions, like the Kelts of Ireland and their druids or the fire worship of the Romans, Germans and Slavs have much in common with the Vedic. Ancient names for the Divine or God, also have their connection. We have divine from Latin deus and Sanskrit deva; Roman Jupiter and Sanskrit Dyaus Pitar; there is Slavic bogu and Vedic bhaga. These reflect a commonality of religious belief and experience, not just a coincidence of language.

While Europe adapted the religious systems of the Middle East it retained its own more richer mythology than these more legalistic religions. That mythology has much in common with the Vedic. It was not only the Greeks who based their culture on the worship of the Sun of inspiration, Apollo; the Vedas worship him similarly as Savitar. Our ancient European ancestors like the older Hindu culture with which they were related, had their own religious beliefs. These were originally quite exalted and aligned with profound occult and Yogic teachings, though they may have degenerated in time. We find remnants of these in the myths and legends of pre-Christian Europe.

Hence, Vedic culture represents an older side of our own western culture. Both ancient Greece and India were highly scientific and intellectual cultures. While Greece turned the mind outward to pursue external realities, India directed its attention within. Yet we find in both the same profound sense of reason, logic, order, harmony, experimentation and experience. We also find a minority in Greece who followed a spiritual view like in India, such as the preSocratics Heraclitus and Parmenides, even much in Plato himself. Similarly we find a minority in India, the Charvakas, who developed a materialistic and scientific view of the world much like the Greeks and rejected all religion as illusion and deception. Ancient India also had republics for a time, like that of ancient Greece.

TOWARDS A GLOBAL CULTURE

The purpose of presenting Hindu and Vedic knowledge is not to impose a religious or cultural belief upon anyone. It is to bring out the universal or spiritual element in human culture. This is, to a great extent, to transcend both religion and culture into the spiritual, the universal. True culture is not a local bias but a local means of approaching the transcendent, a harmonizing ourselves with nature to approach the spiritual power behind her.

Cultures do change. For example, Christianity itself was once seen in Rome as a foreign and eastern religion. Buddhism was long regarded in China as a foreign and western religion. No culture can expect to remain the same without growth or adaptation. The greatest cultures have always been those which have had the greatest openness, which have combined within themselves the greatest diversity of cultural elements, including different races, languages and religions. No culture is homogenous and to the extent a culture tries to be, it usually becomes sterile. To expand one's cultural matrix is not a sign of inferiority but an indication of greatness. A healthy culture is always open to new influences and does not create artificial barriers in knowledge, art or skill. True culture is human and humane, not tied to one special interest group.

Knowledge is not of the north or the south, the east or the west. It is of all time and all places and belongs to all of us. The heritage of all humanity belongs to each human being. Until we are open to that we cannot expect our true humanity to flower. So in approaching the Vedas or any knowledge coming from a different cultural base, we must take its universal and relevant truth. We need not apply it superficially as a fad. We need not imitate it or take it on like a new mask. We need only take from it what communicates to our deeper heart and soul and which is in harmony with the needs of our own situation in life.

On the other hand, we should not merely reject any part of a system of knowledge because at first glance it appears strange or difficult to understand, because it is written in a different language or clothed in a different garb. Nor do we have to be afraid about appearing or thinking differently than the more common influences around us. If we find something that works we should apply it. Hence, outer aspects of Hindu and Vedic culture, like the use of incense or the wearing of white, may also be relevant to us. To adapt them is not necessarily a form of cultural imitation. It may indicate an enhancement of our culture according to influences more in harmony with nature and with the spirit.

There is a simple way wherein we can learn to understand anyone or any culture. This is to not view them as foreign or alien but to accept them as our own, like a forgotten relative, a long lost part of ourselves. It is to endeavor to look at the world through their eyes and with respect for their intelligence. In ancient and modern India this takes the form of treating a guest as form of the Divine, a spiritual friend. We are all human beings, and all human cultures must therefore be fundamentally akin to us, though their forms may appear quite difficult to understand. Behind all culture is the same seeking for love, truth and beauty and wishing to avoid sorrow, strife and poverty.

It is time we stopped making other human beings alien. This only ends up causing enmity and war. If we examine all cultures we find in each all the same basic needs and goals culminating in the search for the Divine or the eternal. A humanity divided against itself cannot stand. Recognizing this we can integrate the world in our own minds. This is the goal of Vedic knowledge. We cannot heal the world without first healing our idea of the world within our mind. To do this we must see the world within us and our self in all aspects of the world. This is to reconstruct the cosmic man who is our true self and embraces all humanity in a single glance.

We live in an era wherein we can explore what is of value in all the world's cultures. It is our duty to extract and use all of them, to cherish all of them, that we might reclaim our global human heritage. Without such a world culture, there can be neither peace in the world nor the flourishing of any part of the world for any significant length of time. We know too well today we are all linked together, that the world is one. We know of immediately what happens in China or Iran, and it can affect us strongly. We can no longer live in one portion of the world and ignore the rest. The divisions of nation and culture must be swept away like the divisions of states and provinces within a country which only recently we have had to go beyond. This is not to deny them their beauty or creative difference but to throw down the artificial boundaries between them. The air does not stop at any national frontier. The sun does not shine differently across the border. We should have at least as much compassion and equanimity as the elements of nature.

There is much more to humanity than our current history tells us. It is hidden in our myths, legends and scriptures. Apart from our chronological history is an invisible or sacred time, the measure of our aspiration for the eternal. In it we find a spiritual humanity seeking the Divine and working for the evolution of consciousness. It is necessary to link up to this greater spiritual sense of the human being to enable us to go beyond the frontiers which have created the present world crisis. It is our connection with it that we find in the Vedas and other ancient teachings.

SPIRITUAL SCIENCE

According to the Yogic and Vedic system the scientific method is not entirely scientific; that is, it is not truly objective and cannot give us knowledge of reality. This may sound like a harsh judgement, and it does not deny the value of science, so let us examine the truth of it. The scientific method is based upon making an assumption, inventing a theory, and then amassing data or making experiments to prove the theory. Whatever we assume we are bound to find facts to prove it; for as Einstein noted, it is the theory that determines what the facts are and where to look for them. While the scientific method may help us understand outer realities, it is not as appropriate for inner realities as it assumes the validity of the outward view.

The Yogic method is quite different. It says first we must empty our mind of all preconceptions, all theories or assumptions and learn to examine things exactly as they are. Then alone can we arrive at knowledge of the thing in itself. This is a matter of meditation. The Yogic method does not start with any presumption whatsoever. It begins with a recognition that we do not really know anything at all because we first of all have not understood ourselves. We have accepted our preconceptions as real without inquiring into their origin, the ego itself. Hence, the Yogic method requires perhaps more doubt and acuity than the scientific method.

Materialistic science is based upon experimentation. Yet as its focus is on the external world, its experiments are with the things outside of ourselves. Its experiments are limited to what has form, to what can be an object of scrutiny for several different observers. We manipulate external objects with various instruments and see what they reveal. As modern science has discovered, such manipulation itself alters the nature of the object and may create the data that it presumes to find.

Spiritual science is also based upon experimentation. Yet, it experiments with the mind itself. It provides us with various methods for observing ourselves and examining how our minds work. It says that if we first do not know ourselves we cannot know anything else, that if we first do not understand our instrument of knowing, the mind, we cannot be certain of the value of the conclusions at which it arrives. The mind has an inherent bias, which is the ego itself and its personal and cultural conditioning. Unless that center is dissolved it must distort the data which comes through it.

Such experiments we can only do for ourselves. Another cannot observe our minds, nor can we look to another to perceive the truth for us. Though such experiments cannot be verified by different observers on the same object like an object in the outer world, they can be verified by different observers examining the same object in their own minds. For example, each of us can observe how anger acts in our minds. While the anger will take different forms, its basic energy and effect will be the same. Such experiments do not alter the objects examined because they involve no motive or manipulation. They are not based on changing the object but seeing it as it is.

Spiritual science does not deny the validity or importance of outer knowledge and experimentation. It does, however, insist upon the priority of the inner knowledge over the outer. Whatever the outer knowledge provides us, it must be within the realm of time. The inner knowledge alone provides us with the means of realizing the eternal, going beyond time. As death is the most inescapable fact of our lives, it behooves us to search out the means of going beyond it. Ultimately, it does not matter if we gain all the outer goals of life like fame, wealth, talent and genius. If we do not know ourselves we are the proverbial man who has gained the world but lost his soul. Spiritual science gives us a way to a knowledge which allows us to know the infinite. If this is possible why should we waste away our lives on the finite?

This spiritual science is not to be confused with false imagination, superstition, with the taking of drugs or artificially induced trances. It is not a matter of wishful thinking but of the most detached inquiry. It demands the utmost seriousness, clarity and objectivity. It requires that we see through the illusions of the mind, the illusions of our self. It regards the mind itself as an illusion and our thought process as a process of illusion building unless we come to understand ourselves. It requires the highest reason and the most consummate intelligence and acuity of perception to uncover the true reality within and around us.

Nor does spiritual science exclude materialistic science. Both have a similar rationality but applied in different directions. Spiritual science only insists that we do not apply the methods of materialistic science to the ultimate issues of life. Materialistic science works through the measurable. The ultimate issues of life — the Divine, the eternal, the infinite, bliss, and freedom — are not measurable and cannot be found by any outward examination. Spiritual science insists that we employ the appropriate instrument to know the truth of a thing. Just as a microscope will not give us a picture of the stars, so an outer oriented science and its machines and computers cannot show us the truth of our inner nature. We cannot find the real man by dissecting our organs or determining the electro-chemical connections in the brain. This is like trying to find the light by taking apart the light bulb. The body is only our shadow. For the ultimate issues we need to know in life; who we are, what life itself is; the appropriate instrument is our own mind directed within, free from attachment or bias to any external or conditioned view. This is the great objectivity of Vedic science.

I have presented in this book, as far as possible, a complete view of Vedic Science — a spiritual science encompassing the whole of life and linking us up to the eternal on all levels. I have outlined its major approaches, not to set them forth in any final manner but to show us how they all fit together. This is to provide us a point of entry into their totality. Many of these approaches have been presented separately in other books and teachings. Most of us probably consider them to be different systems and do not realize their interrelationship. Their connections are a matter of a common origin and tradition. They are not my invention. To understand any of these, it is helpful to know the total picture they are part of.

Spiritual science has an integral structure and a unified world view. It is important to see how each of its aspects fit together and what the relative importance is of each. While we may use aspects of it separately, like following Ayurveda for the physical body, it is important that we do not allow our vision to be fragmented in the process.

Materialistic science is based on analysis and differentiation. Each branch of it tends to become more specialized. It requires its own language and expertise. Proficiency in one branch tends to deny proficiency in the others. For example, a biochemist cannot understand a nuclear physicist.

Spiritual science is the opposite. It is based on synthesis and integration (yoga). Each branch of it tends towards the same universality. Proficiency in one aids in proficiency in the others. For example, an Ayurvedic doctor and a Vedic astrologer have a common system to communicate through. Spiritual science develops out of an integral language and approach. This is the language of the mantra, which is the language of truth perception. It is based on the root principles of the cosmic life like the five elements, the basic energetic realities of nature. Hence, to move from one branch of the spiritual sciences to another requires not the development of a new language but a shifting of the levels on which the same language and logic is applied. It is this openness of the spiritual sciences that can enable a great yogi to be a poet, philosopher, psychologist, doctor, social leader, etc.

The Renaissance idea of the universal man is not false or impossible but requires a different way of knowledge, a different kind of thought. We must return to this synthetic knowledge if we would produce a planetary, global, or cosmic Man. The cosmic human being regards all the Earth as his own, all culture and religion as belonging to himself. He has no artificial or petty barriers of country, culture, race, religion or time that bind his mind. The true knowledge unifies. The capacity of knowledge to bring us together is thereby the test of its validity. May we once more seek that and enshrine it in our hearts as well as our institutions of learning. May such seers, like the rishis of old, arise once more throughout the world!

2

THE ETERNAL TEACHING
SANATANA DHARMA

Many of us in the West are bewildered by this religion we know of as "Hinduism." On one hand, we see the various great yogis and sages of India. They speak of the highest spiritual knowledge and appear to have attained states of consciousness far beyond what our western religions and philosophies have even imagined. They exhibit a state of consciousness which transcends time, place, person, culture, religion, race and all the biases of the human mind and ego. They appear as cosmic beings who have gone beyond the limitations of human life.

These great yogis of India were the first of the eastern teachers to come to the West and to teach meditation. They have also been the first and most prominent to declare the unity of all religions and to thereby move humanity in the direction of a global spiritual path. They have not sought converts but rather have offered ways in which we can enhance our spiritual practice whatever our religious belief may be, or even if we do not have any at all. Their freedom and openness in the spiritual realm we find unparalleled in our experience of our own tradition and rare in other traditions as well.

On the other hand, we can also see the close-minded traditional ethnic Hindu, trapped in caste and culture and addicted to worship of what appear to us as idols. Their narrow attitudes appear opposite that of the great teachers. They appear hidebound in superstition. Through them we tend to see Hinduism as an ethnic religion barred to us and perhaps out of place in the modern world. Much of Hinduism appears in this light as an anachronism, something that was out of date even in the Middle Ages. This is the only side of Hinduism that those in our culture who are not open to the spiritual life can see. Compared to such ethnic Hinduism, Christianity appears enlightened and humane, and modern science and western intellectual culture appears exalted. Given these two sides, what is the truth of this great ancient religion?

The first thing we discover as we inquire into this issue is that the term Hinduism is not found in any of the classical teachings of the so-called Hindu religion. It comes from the Persians and was adapted by the Greeks as a name for the people of India, which they contacted mainly along the banks of the Indus river. Persian Hindu is Greek Indus, the name of a river, nothing more. It is a geographical term.

The religion we call Hinduism is itself largely a religion without a name. It teaches that truth is beyond names and forms and all paths which lead to the Divine are good. As the oldest of religions, the mother of all religions, it accepts all religions. In its long history, going perhaps into prehistoric times, it has seen many other religions come and go. In the scope of its history it saw the great religions of ancient Egypt and Persia, both related to it, rise and fall. It gave birth to many religions including the Buddhist, Jain and Sikh teachings, and it influenced the Muslims, Christians and Taoists. Hence, it does not set itself apart from other religions so much as other religions set themselves apart from it. An educated Hindu has no problem accepting the member of another religion into his own or participating in their religious practices. Hinduism is religion in the generic sense, whereas the others are more like name brands.

As the most tolerant and non-aggressive of all religions Hinduism not only does not try to promote itself, it even allows itself to be given a derogatory name. We would not call Christianity "the Greek religion" or Islam "the Arab religion." Yet we have imposed a geographical term on what is the most complex of all religions. Within the subcontinent of India is one of the greatest diversities of cultures, races and languages in all the world. Though the great majority of these people follow the religion we know of as Hinduism, they are not all alike. They differ much more so than the cultures of Europe, which we would not just simply call "Christian."

Nor was what we call Hinduism ever limited to India much less the banks of the Indus river. Only a few centuries ago it prevailed in Indochina and Indonesia and still has a strong presence in these cultures. The great temple city of Ankor Wat in Cambodia mainly consists of Hindu temples. The island of Bali in Indonesia is still Hindu. Hinduism was often practiced in Afghanistan and Central Asia and Vedic Gods were worshipped in Syria and Turkey in ancient times. While Hinduism never sought converts it allowed itself to grow organically and to spread to many different peoples. It was never simply an ethnic phenomena.

THE DHARMA

The correct name for what we call Hinduism, though seldom used or recognized today, is "Sanatana Dharma," which means literally the "eternal teaching." It is not in essence a defined religion but an openness to spiritual experience. We could also translate it as "the eternally renewed truth;" sanatana not only has the sense of eternity but of perpetual change and renewal. It is also called "Arya Dharma," the teaching of noble people. Buddhism also uses this name, as did the Zoroastrian religion of Persia, both of which are close to the Vedic. Yet this term has been degraded by its usage in Europe by German nationalists and later the Nazis for glorification of their prejudices, and so it is has many wrong and negative conceptions associated with it. Another name for it is "Satya Dharma," the religion of truth.

More simply it is just called the "Dharma;" a Vedic term meaning the law or truth of one's own nature. However, all religions in India have been called the Dharma; Buddhism as the Buddha Dharma, Jainism as the Jain Dharma, the Sikhs as the Sikh Dharma, etc. These we can put under the greater umbrella of "Dharmic traditions" which we can see as Hinduism or the spiritual traditions of India in the broadest sense. All these dharmic traditions teach Yoga, meditation and aim at self-realization. They have perhaps more in common with each other than do the different sects within Christianity.

HINDUISM

By modern usage and convenience we can still apply the name Hinduism to this Vedic or eternal Dharma. We should, however, realize that it can be a misnomer. To understand it better we will refer to it in this book mainly as the Vedic or Yogic teaching, this being its inner or spiritual side. It is to its universal essence and capacity to renew itself that we look to here, not merely its forms from the past. It is to the fire that we look, not to the embers or the ashes.

Hinduism consists of many different sects and teachings, much more so than any other religion. It is not so much a religion in particular as a compendium of religious and spiritual teachings. It has no overall one messiah, one prophet, saviour or great teacher. It has no single bible or scripture. Its ultimate scripture is the Divine word within the heart. Its savior is the Divine within man (which is the meaning of Narayana, the name of Vishnu as the saviour). There is no standard practice. It is not centered on any single name or form of the Divine. There is no set lineage or network of teachers for all to follow. It contains within itself all the different approaches to the Divine used by humanity since the dawn of history, from some of the apparently most primitive to the highest. It allows for the worship of the Divine in all forms; Gods and Goddesses of every kind, with all possible human and animal representations.

Yet it also teaches that the Divine is beyond form, is our very Self. It is the proverbial elephant which we as blind men tend to take only one part of as the whole. We find many opposites combined within its great scope.

In its tradition are many teachers, with many who have realized the Divine within their own consciousness. Usually each individual will follow his own teacher or guru rather than any standard prophet. The emphasis on the guru is on this direct and personal connection with the Divine. The real guru, of whom the outer teacher is only a representative, is our own inner Self. Once we are connected with our inner being we go beyond all outer teachers or teachings.

Actually, Hinduism is not a religion at all in the ordinary sense of the word. It is an expression of the natural religion, the religion of life. It teaches that each of us should have our own religion. It encourages freedom, spontaneity, and individuality in our approach to the Divine and says that religion is a private and personal, not a public and social matter — a matter of the heart, not a badge we wear or a title we take. It teaches that the individual is God — you are God. It says that whatever way we approach the Divine will not work until we recognize the Divinity within ourselves. It does not make us subordinate to Christ, Buddha, Krishna, Mohammed or any other great figure but insists that we ourselves are as much the Divine as any other human being and until we realize that we live in illusion.

Hence, we could say it is the religion of individualism rather than a collective or group belief as most religions tend to be. It is the least organized of all religions. It borders on anarchism and allows almost anything which expresses an attempt to reach the Divine or the source of things. Thus it is the religion most in harmony with the individual who wishes to go beyond organized belief. In this respect it is the most global of all religions because it can be adapted to any individual of any time or place, any religious or non-religious background, without any violation of their nature.

Hindu children are not indoctrinated in any religion but allowed to choose their spiritual path from the great diversity the religion offers or even outside of that if they wish. Hinduism emphasizes choosing and following a path, not what path we should follow.

Hinduism is more a set of tools for religious practice rather than a doctrine one must follow or a faith in which one must believe. It includes polytheistic, pantheistic, monotheistic, monistic and nontheistic teachings. It includes all the Yogic approaches of knowledge, devotion, technique and service. Its form has constantly changed throughout the centuries, yet without denying the validity of the earlier teachings.

It is not a religion that was given once in a definitive form. It is not based on a single historical event or revelation, like the birth of Christ or the ascension of Mohammed. It has no final revelation but a continuous stream of living experience. Its emphasis is more on modern teachers who have realized the truth in a way we can understand today, rather than on following some set example from bygone ages. Its tradition is constantly being adapted to the present. For this reason adapting the Vedic and Yogic teaching to the West does not require we become Hindus or limit ourselves to any particular religion. We may use its tools in the practice of any religion or we can use them directly in the spiritual life without any religious belief. It does require, however, that we adapt the tools of Yoga to the needs of our individual nature and the Divine presence within us. That is entering the true path and becoming conscious of our role in the universal religion which is life itself.

THE CULTURE OF THE DHARMA

This, however, does not mean that it is wrong for us to adapt some of the cultural or outer forms of Yoga. Outer aspects of the teaching like the diet or the style of art may be relevant for enhancing our lives. While we need not look or dress or act like Hindus we need not go to the other extreme and reject the culture of Yoga so as not to appear different than our neighbors. Wearing white, for example, can elevate and purify the mind. To use such practices may not be a blind adaptation of a foreign culture but based on an understanding of the spiritual reason beyond the cultural form. As such it will serve to universalize our culture, not to limit it.

As its foundation Hinduism possesses a broad and complete cultural matrix. It has its own language, poetry, drama, dance, art, sculpture, science, mathematics and medicine. Christianity relies upon primarily a Greco-Roman influence for the intellectual or secular part of its culture, like art and philosophy. Islam relies to a great extent on ancient Greek and Persian sources. Buddhism relies primarily on other sources in the same way; the Tibetans taking much of Hindu culture like art and medicine, as did the Indian Buddhists, the Chinese Buddhists following the earlier Taoist and Chinese culture. Hinduism alone of the world's major religions is primarily self-based and self-reliant in both the inner and outer aspects of life and culture. It provides a rich and open field for the soul to grow with much to use on all levels. Its very richness is often its difficulty as there are in it so many paths to choose from, so many levels of participation, that it is possible to be led astray by secondary concerns or interests. Such a great cultural field is important for a creative and spiritual global culture.

Hence, behind the Yogic teaching is the whole Sanatana Dharma or eternal religion and its legacy of spiritual practices from all time. In addition the culture of the Dharma is useful in all spheres of our life. What is important is for us to continue that stream and use it in a creative way.

This is neither to blindly follow or reject it. It is neither to become caught in its forms nor to fail to see their message. Vedic and Yogic science, therefore, are part of a religion and a culture. They are in fact the basis of all religion and culture. While their essence is in the spiritual their relevance is to the whole of life, and it is to that complete picture of them we address ourselves here.

THE RELIGION OF TRUTH

In reality there is only one religion, as there is only one truth. The names and forms of religions are but appearances or perhaps distortions of that one truth. It is wrong to take them too seriously or to think that any one of them could ever triumph or should ever be promoted against the others. The true religion is also not a matter of numbers. It is not important how many people join it. One practitioner of the truth of any great religion is worth thousands of mere followers.

What matters is how much we live up to that quality of truth which is not deceived by temporary appearances. No one can really join this universal religion or leave it. The true religion is being itself. If we do not live in truth to that extent we cease to be truly religious. If we live in truth, we see the sacred nature of all life, we fulfill all religions which have been or are to be. Religion, therefore, requires no dilemma or choice. It only requires that we be who we are and as we are, that we come from our true heart rather than seek to project an appearance or maintain some form in the outer world.

Just as no group can dispense or rule over life, just as nobody owns the air, just as no group of artists can claim to own art, so can no one claim to possess truth or govern the religious lives of others. It is time we dispensed with trying to judge the religious and spiritual life of people by the names, forms and numbers of the outer world. We must take such political, geographical and cultural barriers out of the realm of inner seeking, whose only real purpose is to connect us with the infinite. Without this our inner life is an hypocrisy, a reflection of political or social biases.

This religion of truth is not a thing of one life or our identity created within one incarnation. It is the real project of our soul from life to life. It is not one part of life but the essence and totality of our entire being in all our lives. Hence, it sees the religions of this world as mere shadows of the religion of our soul which transcends time. It addresses our needs as souls from incarnation to incarnation in the many different levels of unfoldment of our spiritual nature. It does not stop short at the appearances present in our current world context. It also teaches when relevant our connection with other worlds more subtle than the physical.

It is this religion of truth which is emphasized here. It is not an organized belief but the emergence of consciousness. It has its order in life but an order which unfolds the creative and spiritual potentials of life, not one which casts a shadow over our heart. To enter into this stream of consciousness is not simply to take upon a new identity or role in the outer life. It is to step outside of the realm of images and roles. To follow this order is not to impose some rule or authority upon ourselves but to come into harmony with the rhythm of our own inner being.

If there is truth in this, let it be adopted as we can. If there is no truth in this then let it be discarded as we wish. Truth always wins in the end, not untruth, as the Upanishads say. Though the present moment may belong to the forces of ignorance, to the truth belongs all eternity and all time must bow down before it.

The measure of who we are in life is not how much we own or how people regard us. It is what portion of the eternal we have discovered in life, as that alone goes with us at death. The eternal is the universal and it is through discovering it and enshrining it again within us that our journey proceeds.

3
NATURE'S MEDICINE
AYURVEDA

Ayurveda is the knowledge or science, veda, of life or longevity, ayur. It is the medical aspect of Vedic science and regarded as an Upaveda, or secondary Vedic system. Today it is perhaps the most commonly known of the Vedic sciences. In the Vedic and Yogic system health is seen as a basis for creative and spiritual growth, not as an end in itself. The goal of life is not just to live but to find the meaning of life. Hence, we should use the time and energy our health provides for developing our higher nature. Thus Ayurveda naturally leads to the other and deeper aspects of Vedic knowledge.

Ayurveda is an aspect of Yoga and is most allied with Hatha Yoga, the Yoga of the physical body, with which it can be combined. While Hatha Yoga provides us the exercises for physical health, flexibility and the dissolution of tension, Ayurveda gives the knowledge of how to care for our body in terms of diet and medicine. Both serve as means of harmonizing the physical body so that the powers of our inner consciousness can come into action through it. While the body is not the goal of the spiritual or creative life, it is the foundation. Without health we cannot do anything in life. Hence, Ayurveda is of importance to all.

Ayurveda is the medicine of nature, the medicine of life. It does not give us a set of theoretical principles to impose upon our biological functioning. Rather it seeks to present to the human mind the principles and powers of Nature herself. It teaches us to put into practice Nature's great principles of health and natural living. For this reason it employs the language of nature; an energetic system of the elements and biological humors, a simple yet profound system of correspondences, not a complex scientific, materialistic or biochemical terminology.

It considers that it is more important to know what aspect of nature is working within us; for example, if there is too much or too little heat in our system, rather than to be able to describe this dysfunction in terms of pathogens or biochemical malfunctions. Its terms, therefore, the biological humors, the elements and their qualities, do not originate from conceptual thought or scientific experiments but through direct observation of Nature herself. They represent the powers of Nature working within us, the great Gods or cosmic powers of the vital or life-plane to whom we must do homage (i.e., respect and follow their laws). Just as we have the powers of water, fire and wind working in the environment around us, they work on a biological level within us. Just as allowing a fire to get too close will burn us externally, allowing our inner fire to burn too highly will damage our internal organs.

Ayurveda is a form of naturalistic medicine or naturopathy. According to its wisdom it is Nature herself that heals. All we can do is assist in her process by attuning ourselves to her movements. Therefore, Ayurveda emphasizes the balancing of the life-force within us as the basis of all treatment. Ayurveda is based on diet and herbs for its treatment but uses many specially prepared mineral substances as well. It provides us with a complete life-regime through an integrated science of life-style counseling that deals with body and mind, and with both the individual and society. Its goal is not to suppress our symptoms but to give us the tools to understand our nature and live in harmony with it.

SELF-HEALING

For this reason, Ayurveda is primarily a system of self-healing. It tells us that what we do for ourselves is more important in correcting our condition than what others may do for us. As the responsibility for creating our condition comes from us, so too must be the responsibility for rectifying it.

Ayurveda states that how we live everyday is more significant in determining our health than what we do once in a while. An occasional visit to a doctor or health spa to improve our health cannot correct the effects of a long term wrong diet or stressful living. What we eat everyday is more important than what pill or vitamin we take once in a while to compensate for it.

According to Ayurveda we cannot expect to get well through natural healing methods if our lives themselves are out of harmony with Nature. For this reason, it cannot be used as a palliative measure to maintain our artificial and stressful life-styles. Ayurveda may not help us to continue on as we have been but may insist upon a real change in our manner of living if we wish to really get well.

As a spiritually based medicine, it tells us that psychological and spiritual factors usually outweigh physical factors in causing diseases. Hence even if we follow the right physical regimes, if our emotions are disturbed or if we have no real spiritual purpose in life, we cannot expect to truly heal. We cannot cure the body apart from the mind, or the mind apart from the soul. To treat diseases on only a physical level deals with the effects, not the causes, and cannot address the major part of the problem.

We cannot cheat Nature or fool life. Short cuts, easy fixes, quick cures, wishful thinking, magic remedies and panaceas are not part of Ayurveda. Life demands a tremendous integrity, self-discipline and self-awareness to take us beyond disease and sorrow. Ayurveda may not make things easier for us in the short term but in the long run it allows us to open up to the real energy of the cosmic life within us and to assume responsibility for our own existence. There is a magic in Ayurveda, but it is the magic of consciousness and moment by moment right action. Its magic is not that it takes us off the hook by solving our problems for us but that it gives us the right tools to effectively and finally dissolve them.

ACTIVE AND PASSIVE THERAPIES

There are two forms of therapies: what could be called active and passive. A passive therapy is what someone else does to us. An active therapy is what we participate in or do for ourselves. Active therapies are always stronger than passive ones. Passive therapies may be necessary in acute conditions but they cannot of themselves bring about real change.

Our culture itself is excessively passive. We are largely spectators observing others perform. We let others live our lives and we in turn watch them on the sidelines or in front of the screen. Our lives have very little direct experience or creative involvement, which according to Yoga is the only really liberating or fulfilling factor in life. We let other people tell us what to do, how to think, who we are, where to go, what to buy. We let others fix our food, entertain us, tell us how to make love, tell us what God is and so on. In the same way we let the medical establishment run our health. We follow the idea of health which others give us, not what we experience for ourselves or discover to be true and effective in our own lives. If we become the victims of this process there is no one to blame but ourselves. Just as no one can breathe for us, no one can make us healthy or happy.

Ayurveda holds that there is no real healer, no magical doctor or magical pill. The magic is in us, in arousing our own life-force and connecting with our own soul, the source of life. No machine can give us life, nor can mechanical tests really measure the life-force within us which is the true measure of our health. Medical diagnoses may be more harmful than helpful if they do not acknowledge the ability of the life-force to overcome all diseases. The diagnosis of cancer, for example, often tends to destroy the life will in the patient and thereby prevents any cure from taking place.

No substance we take from the outside can be anything more than a catalyst. We, each of us individually, have to learn what our nature really is and through it how to live in harmony with the cosmic life. No one can do this for us, and as long as we are unwilling to do so we must contract disease. For this reason Ayurveda is a constitutional or individually oriented medicine. It has no form of mass treatment or mass diagnosis. It is opposed to all standardized medicine. It says that each individual is different, and even if their diseases are apparently the same we still cannot treat them in the same way.

Those looking for mere comfort or for someone to make them healthy without their own effort may find Ayurveda limited or unhelpful. But it is the most honest form of medicine and the one which does not take power over us. If we begin to apply its tools in our own lives we will get great results but only if we do so in harmony with Nature and through the course of time with the appropriate adjustments to the rhythms of life.

THE BACKGROUND OF AYURVEDA

Ayurveda has its complex clinical methods including surgery and the use of strong medications. These, however, are secondary to its primary self-healing approach. Its eight branches are: internal medicine (kayachikitsa), surgery (shalyatantra), diseases of the head (shalakya-tantra), pediatrics (kaumarabhritya), toxicology (agadatantra), psychiatry (bhutavidya), rejuvenation (rasayana) and revitalization (vajikarana).

Ayurveda, as typical of the Vedic sciences, is applied differently by its various practitioners as it also emphasizes creative intelligence, not a standardized approach. It does not present us with just one way of looking at health or disease but gives us a whole spectrum in harmony with the vastness of life. Hence, it cannot be understood from a purely scientific, intellectual or materialistic perspective.

Ayurveda is based upon the spiritual and psychological background of Yoga, Sankhya and Vedanta. From these come its methods for healing the mind. It holds that diseases are of two causes; either owing to imbalances of energies in the body itself or owing to karmic, that is psychological causes. The latter are thought to predominate over the former, though both factors are present in most diseases.

The three main classical texts for Ayurveda are *Charak, Sushrut,* and *Vagbhat.* While they are still studied today and give the fundamental principles, much of their material is no longer relevant, so many modern books have been written to adapt them to changing conditions. While the form we find these texts in today was not finalized until the early centuries A.D., *Charak* and *Sushrut* are about the same time as Krishna (c. 1500-1000 B.C.). Many Ayurvedic practices are also mentioned in Buddhist teachings and in the stories of the Buddha himself. Ayurveda was adapted by the Buddhists and is the basis of Buddhist medicine. Vagbhat himself was a Buddhist, and his text and commentaries on it are still commonly studied in Buddhist medicine. Nagarjuna, the most famous of the Buddhist siddhas, and perhaps the most renowned figure in the Mahayana Buddhist tradition after the Buddha, was a great Ayurvedic doctor. From him originate many of the special mineral or alchemical preparations (rasas) still prepared and used in India today. Tibetan medicine thus is also predominately Ayurvedic with a mixture of Chinese influence.

The older Greek medicine used in Europe until the seventeenth century and still used in Islamic countries and by the Muslims of India (called Unnani medicine) is very similar to Ayurveda. It employs a four humor rather than a three humor model. In India, Ayurvedic and Unnani forms of medicine are commonly practised together. Hence, Ayurvedic knowledge has had a broad application and remains relevant to the main natural healing traditions in the world.

Ayurveda in its origins is an integral part of the most ancient *Rig Veda*. The three main Vedic Gods, Indra, Agni and Soma, relate to the three Doshas or biological humors of Ayurveda as Vata (air), Pitta (fire) and Kapha (water). Indra has the energy of air and the life-force and is often equated with it as Vata or Vayu. Agni is the essential energy of fire and Soma, the essential energy of water. The Vedic chants provide the sound vibrations which balance the three humors in the body and open up their subtle potentials in the mind. From them a complete mantra therapy for disease can be derived.

THE BIOLOGICAL HUMORS
THE THREE DOSHAS

According to Ayurveda, the human body is ruled by three fundamental life-forces: Vata, Pitta and Kapha. These are often translated as wind, bile and phlegm. Vata is also often called the biological air-humor, Pitta the biological fire-humor and Kapha the biological water-humor.

The humors are called Doshas in Sanskrit, meaning what spoils or causes decay, as they are not only the forces which produce and sustain the body in their normal condition but those which, when out of balance, serve to destroy it. Death is inherent in life. Even our normal process of metabolism is not only growing new cells but causing old cells to die and be discarded. Growth and life must eventually turn into decay and death. Health in the body thus consists in the right balance of the creative and destructive forces of the Doshas.

Each of the biological humors is composed of two elements; the first which provides for its primary force, the second which gives a medium for its manifestation. Vata consists of air and ether; air is its active side and ether or space its medium or field of movement. Pitta consists of fire and water; fire is its active side, water or oil is its field of combustion as fire cannot exist directly in the body without destroying it. Kapha consists of water and earth; water is its active force and earth its container.

Yet the biological humors are not the same as the elements. They are forms of the life-force working through and animating the elements. They are different aspects of the soul. The elements in themselves are inanimate. They are never really alive but can be activated by the biological humors, like a wire is by an electric current. This life force is reflected from the soul, our eternal being, upon the physical body by the lens of the mind. Hence, embodied life is always temporary. What comes from the inanimate elements and is formed of them must return to them. Similarly, the life-force which comes from the eternal must eventually return to it. The current of life eventually must wear out the wire of the body. Nevertheless, life can still be prolonged far beyond its ordinary limits, and Ayurveda gives us many keys to this process.

Vata is dry, light, cold, rough, subtle and agitated in qualities. It is the root of the humors, tissues and waste materials of the body. In its natural state it sustains effort, inhalation, exhalation, movement, the discharge of impulses, the equilibrium of the tissues and the coordination of the senses.

Pitta is oily, penetrating, hot, light, unpleasant in odor, mobile and liquid. It governs digestion, thermogenesis, visual perception, hunger, thirst, lustre, complexion, understanding, intelligence, courage and softness of the body.

Kapha is wet, cold, heavy, slow, sticky, soft and firm in qualities. It gives stability, lubrication, holding together of the joints and such qualities as patience, calm and devotion.

CONSTITUTIONAL TYPES

The biological humors as the predominant forces in our body become the main factors which determine our psycho-physical constitution. According to Ayurveda we are not all alike physically nor do our bodies react in the same way. Each of us is a unique combination and proportion of the biological humors.

Hence, Ayurveda generally divides individuals into three types relative to the predominance of the three humors in their nature, as Vata, Pitta or Kapha. From these, seven basic types are distinguished, pure Vata, pure Pitta, pure Kapha, dual Vata-Pitta, dual Pitta-Kapha, dual Kapha-Vata and a balanced, triple or Vata-Pitta-Kapha type.

Some Ayurvedic doctors give numbers to represent the proportion of Vata, Pitta and Kapha in the body or in the disease process, like Vata 4, Pitta 2, Kapha 1, showing a high Vata state. But there is no standard way of doing this, and each practitioner may do it differently.

Vata

Vata people, those in whom the biological air-humor predominates, are said to be unusually tall or short, thin, bony, with prominent veins, and generally poor tissue development. Their complexion may be dull or lacking in lustre, with possible brown or dark discolorations, with dry or cracked skin. They possess variable appetites, tend toward constipation or hard stool, have scanty sweat or urination, are intolerant of cold and wind and, though they have immediate energy, have low endurance and stamina.

Vata types are nervous, restless, hyperactive, excitable and may suffer from insomnia or disturbed sleep. They are changeable, curious and adaptable, with sensitive and quick minds and reflexes, are often talkative and can be absent minded. They tend towards insecurity, fear and anxiety when emotionally out of balance, can be easily disturbed and are prone to worry.

Pitta

Pitta people, those in whom the biological fire-humor is highest, are average or moderate in build and height, with good muscles. They have good circulation, warm and oily skin, ruddy complexions with possible redness of face or eyes, with delicate hair and possible early greying or balding. They have sharp appetites, much thirst and sweat easily. They tend toward loose elimination and profuse urination and commonly have yellow discoloration of the stool or urine. They are intolerant of heat and sun and may to bleed easily.

Pitta types are aggressive, dominating, with leadership potentials, good speakers and workers. They are critical, perceptive, intelligent and have sharp memories. They tend toward irritability and anger when emotionally out of balance and are prone to conflict and argument.

Kapha

Kapha people, those of the biological water-humor, tend towards overweight, are stocky or well built with good development of tissues. They have white, pale and moist skin, abundant and thick hair and large eyes. They have constant appetites but slow metabolism and are intolerant of cold and damp. They have abundant bodily secretions and often have too much mucus in their systems. They are slow in movement and find it difficult to get going but possess good endurance and generally strong immune systems.

Kapha types are calm, stable, devoted, loyal with slow but steady minds and memory. They may suffer from lethargy, lack of motivation or excess sleep. Their emotional imbalances are toward greed, attachment and depression. They can be possessive or sentimental.

***

We should remember in the delineations of the three types that their excess features are exaggerated for purposes of identification. No one of them is necessarily better or worse than the others. What is important is to live in harmony with our nature and its higher potentials, not to try to change it.

Each type tends towards certain diseases. Vata types tend towards nervous system disorders, anxiety attacks, insomnia, arthritis, and constipation. Most wasting diseases and diseases of old age are of a Vata nature. Vata has the greatest number of diseases because, as the most fundamental of the biological humors its imbalances can have greater consequences.

Pitta tends towards fever, infection, inflammatory diseases, hyperacidity, ulcers, skin rashes, bleeding disorders, and liver problems. Kapha has congestive disorders, colds, flus, bronchitis, pneumonia and diseases of edema and excess water. Though each type may get any disease, each tends more toward diseases of its same qualities.

One of the humors when high can damage the others as well. For example, high Kapha can clog the channels and the nerves and cause epilepsy or strokes, thus resulting in Vata disorders.

It is important that we know our individual constitution and how to deal with it. Ayurveda prescribes diet, herbs and life-style per constitution. Generally, we can all do well with a sattvic life-style, with pure, natural vegetarian food, and peaceful, compassionate and humane living. When out of balance, however, we should always consider diet and herbs according to the deranged humor. For this we should consult an Ayurvedic practitioner.

AYURVEDIC ANATOMY AND PHYSIOLOGY

Ayurveda has its own system of anatomy and physiology considering not only the gross body but also the currents of life-force and connections with the subtle body. It recognizes five different types, each of Vata, Pitta and Kapha according to their different sites and functions in the body.

The Seven Tissues (Sapta Dhatu)

Ayurveda views the body as the development of seven tissues. These are plasma, blood, muscle, fat, bone, marrow and nerve tissue and reproductive tissue (rasa, rakta, mamsa, meda, asthi, majja and shukra in Sanskrit). They form a concentric circle from the gross to the subtle. Those more gross nourish those more subtle, which in turn serve to support those more gross. Diseases of the deeper tissues, like nerve and bone, are usually much worse than those of the superficial, like plasma and blood.

The Channel Systems (Srotas)

Fourteen channel systems are recognized in Ayurveda, with sixteen in the female. They are similar to the meridian systems in Chinese medicine but include most of our physiological systems as well.

Three exist to bring nutrients into the body. These are the channel systems of breath, food and water. Seven exist to support the seven tissues. Three exist to eliminate waste-materials from the body, the systems of the feces, urine and sweat.

The mind is a special system in itself connecting to the nervous and reproductive systems.

The female contains two special systems, those of menstruation and lactation, which operate alternatively.

Diseases are classified according to the humors, tissues and channels systems they effect.

THE SIX TASTES

Ayurveda recognizes six tastes in food and herbs. These are: sweet, salty, sour, pungent, bitter and astringent. Each is composed of two elements. Sweet is composed of earth and water; salty of water and fire; sour of earth and fire; pungent of fire and air; bitter of air and ether; and astringent of earth and air.

Sweet is sweet or pleasant in taste as in most foods such as sugars, starches, carbohydrates, dairy, nuts, and meat. It is strengthening and nourishing and has a tonic, demulcent and laxative effect. Salty is as in table salt. It has a stimulant, demulcent, laxative and sedative effect. Sour is as in sour fruit, pickles or vinegar. It has a stimulant, expectorant and laxative effect. Pungent is as in spices like pepper, mustard, ginger or cinnamon. Its properties are stimulant, diaphoretic, decongestant, analgesic and diuretic. Bitter is as in bitters like gentian, and golden seal. Its action is cleansing, detoxifying, alterative and diuretic. Astringent is as in unripe bananas, persimmons or herbs with tannins like alum root, witch hazel or oak bark. Its effect is to stop excess discharges and is astringent, hemostatic, vulnerary, expectorant and diuretic in action.

Three tastes increase and three tastes decrease each of the biological humors. They are increased by those tastes which predominate in the same elements which compose them, and they are decreased by those which are of different or opposite nature than the elements which compose them.

Kapha is increased by sweet, salty and sour (which predominate in earth and water) and decreased by pungent, bitter and astringent (which predominate in air). Vata is decreased by sweet, salty and sour and increased by bitter, astringent and pungent. Pitta is increased by pungent, sour and salty (which predominate in fire) and decreased by bitter, astringent and sweet (which have no fire).

TREATMENT METHODS

Ayurvedic treatment methods are of two kinds: constitutional or clinical. Constitutional remedies include diet, mild herbs and proper life-style per constitution. Clinical remedies consist of strong herbs and medications and Pancha Karma.

Generally, all therapies are divided into two types: tonification or reduction. Tonification therapy, also called supplementation, is indicated for the weak, debilitated, convalescent, emaciated, pregnant, very young or very old. It rebuilds our internal energy and brings about increase of the tissues but may not clear up toxins. Reduction therapy is indicated in acute diseases. It eliminates disease-causing factors and pathogens but may have a depleting effect upon the body. Both methods may be combined or used alternatively. Generally, tonification follows reduction, as cleansing allows us to rebuild the body on a higher level.

Tonification consists of rich diet, tonic and strengthening herbs, adequate rest and relaxation, avoidance of excessive activity or stimulation. Reduction methods are twofold as preliminary or radical. Preliminary or mild reduction therapies (shamana) consist of light eating or fasting, herbs to improve digestion, massage, sweating therapy and proper exercise. Radical reduction (shodhana) consists of Pancha Karma, strongly reducing herbs, drugs or surgery.

Pancha Karma

Pancha Karma means the five purification or cleansing practices. It is the main cleansing method in Ayurveda. Its methods are purgation (virechana), medicated enemas (basti), therapeutic vomiting (vamana), nasal medications (nasya) and therapeutic release of toxic blood (rakta moksha). Purgation is most useful for Pitta, medicated enemas for Vata and therapeutic vomiting for Kapha.

To aid in this process preliminary cleansing methods are done to bring the aggravated humors to the digestive tract for their elimination from the body. These are oil therapy (snehana) and steam therapy (svedana). Oil therapy consists of massage with medicated oils. Steam therapy involves use of a sweat box or directing the steam through hoses (nadi sveda). In Pancha Karma three weeks of such methods may be given. Modern short term version of Pancha Karma may last only a few days, but their results may be limited.

Some Pancha Karma centers are opening in this country. Pancha Karma provides the most effective Ayurvedic clinical method for treating or preventing disease. It is important, however, to preceed it with the right diet and cleansing preparation and to follow it up with the right life-style and rejuvenation medications. Otherwise, its effects will not be lasting.

Ayurvedic Massage and Marma Therapy

Ayurvedic massage relies heavily on the oil and steam treatments that accompany Pancha Karma. Yet it can be applied apart from Pancha Karma to treat many different conditions. Ayurvedic massage emphasizes the use of medicated oils externally, specially prepared by cooking powerful herbs in the oil base. Such oils provide a nutrition to the skin and through the skin to the muscles, bones and nerves, which otherwise cannot be gained.

Like the acupuncture points of Chinese medicine, Ayurveda also has its sensitive marma points. These points can be treated by massage, herbs, aromatic oils or the application of heat and thereby can aid in balancing the energy flow in the body and cure disease.

SOME IMPORTANT AYURVEDIC FOODS

Almonds	Nourishes the lungs, the reproductive system and nerve tissue; gives strength, stops cough; is an expectorant; is excellent for Vata.
Basmati Rice	Nourishing, harmonizing, and balancing to all tissues and organs.
Chyavan Prash	Ayurvedic tonic herbal jelly prepared with Amla; good source of vitamin C; builds all tissues and organs and strengthens the immune system.
Coconut	Nourishes the lungs and skin, relieves fever and thirst; good for Pitta.
Curry	Combination of spices, usually with a base of turmeric to aid digestion and increase the strengthening power of foods.
Ghee	(Clarified butter) Nourishes the liver, nerves and brain; relieves fever and infection; best for Pitta.

Honey	Expectorant, laxative, tonic, and rejuvenative; best sweetener for Kapha; aids in weight reduction.
Jaggery or Gur	(Raw sugar, a similar type is sold in this country as sucanet.) Builds all body tissues; warming; good for Vata.
Kicharee	A combination of mung, basmati rice and spices; an excellent food for convalescence or detoxification.
Milk	Nourishes all tissues, cools and calms the mind and heart, stops bleeding, aphrodisiac, and laxative; good for Pitta and Vata.
Mung Beans	Nourishes and cleanses the blood and liver, clears fevers, infections and toxins, aids in convalescence and rejuvenation, and balances metabolism.
Mustard Oil	Light, warm oil good for preventing overweight.
Papaya	Nourishing and thirst-relieving, promotes menstruation, and aids digestion.
Pineapple	Cleanses the blood and liver, aids digestion, and good for Pitta.
Pomegranate	Builds the blood, stops bleeding, astringent, antacid, and good for Pitta and Kapha.
Rock Salt	Best salt for improving digestion.
Sesame Seeds	Builds all the organs and tissues, improves growth of bone, teeth, hair, and excellent for Vata.
Yogurt	Strengthening to all tissues, astringent, and good for Vata.

IMPORTANT AYURVEDIC HERBS

Ayurveda has many important herbs, including special powerful tonics, rejuvenatives and restoratives to the immune system, much like Chinese medicine.

Aloe	(Aloe vera) Tonic to the liver and spleen, laxative, emmenagogue, alterative, detoxifying, and excellent for Pitta.
Amalaki	(Emblica officinalis) Tonic, rejuvenative, laxative, builds the blood, and good for all types.

Arjuna	(Terminalia arjuna) Tonic and restorative to the heart, alterative, hemostatic, and promotes healing of tissues.
Ashwagandha	(Withania somnifera) A good tonic to the brain, reproductive system and bones; analgesic and sedative to the mind but without depressant effect: excellent for Vata.
Bala	(Sida cordifolia) Tonic to the lungs and reproductive system; gives strength; for Pitta and Vata.
Black Musali	(Curculigo orchiodes) Tonic, stimulant, antirheumatic, and good for Vata.
Bibhitaki	(Terminalia baelerica) Tonic, astringent, expectorant, and good for Kapha and the lungs.
Calamus	(Acorus calamus) Nervine, expectorant, stimulant, stomachic; excellent for improving intelligence and speech; for Kapha and Vata.
Castor Oil	Purgative, good for nervous and arthritic disorders.
Coriander	(Coriandrum sativum) Digestive stimulant, antiallergy, and diuretic; best spice for Pitta.
Garlic	(Allium sativa) Tonic, stimulant, expectorant, antibiotic, and rejuvenative; for Vata and Kapha.
Gotu Kola	(Centella asiatica) Tonic to the brain and liver, sedative, alterative, diuretic, and hemostatic; improves intelligence, and good for meditation.
Guduchi	(Tinospora cordifolia) Tonic, antipyretic, alterative, good for chronic infectious diseases, weak immune systems and lingering fevers.
Guggul	(Commiphora mukul) Expectorant, analgesic, and alterative; excellent medicine for arthritis, gout, diabetes, and obesity.
Haritaki	(Terminalia chebula) Tonic to the brain and colon; astringent, laxative, and excellent for Vata.
Jatamansi	(Nardostachys jatamansi) Nervine, tonic, and calmative.
Kapikacchu	(Mucuna pruriens) Tonic and aphrodisiac to the reproductive system; rejuvenative; excellent for Vata.

Phyllanthus niruri	(Bhumyamalaki) Liver tonic, alterative, and chola-gogue; for Pitta and Kapha.
Saffron	(Crocus sativa) Stimulant, emmenagogue, aphrodis-iac, good for heart, liver, spleen and female reproduc-tive system.
Shankha Pushpi	(Canscora decussata) Nervine tonic.
Shatavari	(Asparagus racemosus) Good tonic to the lymph, blood and female reproductive system; nourishing to the heart; for Pitta and Vata.
Shilajit	Tonic, rejuvenative, and diuretic; excellent for diabe-tes; strengthens kidneys; excellent for Kapha.
Turmeric	(Curcuma longa) Stimulant, alterative, astringent, an-titumor, and antibiotic; good for the skin and for com-plexion; promotes healing; best general spice.
White Musali	(Asparagus adscendens) Tonic, demulcent, and aphro-disiac; like shatavari.

AYURVEDIC PREPARATIONS

Anjan	Ayurvedic ointments.
Arishta & Asava	Ayurvedic herbal wines.
Avaleha & Prash	Herbal jellies and confections.
Bhasma	Specially prepared mineral ashes.
Churna	Herbal powders.
Ghrita	Medicated ghee.
Guggul	Herbal preparations in myrrh like resin base.
Guti & Vati	Herbal pills.
Hima	Cold infusion.
Kalka	Herbal paste.
Kvath	Decoction.
Phant	Hot infusion.
Rasa	Alchemical preparations in purified mercury/sulfur base.
Svarasa	Fresh juice of herbs.
Taila	Medicated sesame oil.

REJUVENATION AND IMMORTALITY (RASAYANA)

We all seek immortality. It is our natural desire to want to live forever. According to the Vedas, this desire is misplaced. Immortality is the natural quality of the soul. The mortal body has as its property eventual decay and death. The mortal can never become immortal, and the immortal can never become mortal. Nothing can change its nature. It is only because we identify ourselves with the physical body that we wish for it to live forever and see in its demise the end of our existence. Immortality always belongs to us in our true nature as an eternal conscious being.

While Ayurveda does not believe in physical immortality, it does hold that our lives are much shorter than they need to be, owing to our inharmonious living patterns. It maintains that long life is a good general goal, as the more time we have in an incarnation the more karma we can work through. Assumption of a new body is not only a difficult process, but it is a challange to retain our spiritual purpose in each incarnation. For this reason Ayurveda teaches us several means of prolonging life.

The methods of prolonging life, however, are not methods of avoiding death. Life can only be renewed through death. Ayurvedic rejuvenation methods allow us to undergo a mini-death process in body and mind to allow for rejuvenation. If we are not willing to die psychologically to our attachment to the past and our ego identity, these practices seldom work. Hence, they all involve cleansing and purification.

More important than rejuvenation of the body is rejuvenation of the mind. Our brain cells get old under the burden of memory. To reach true awareness in old age it is necessary to cleanse the cells of these memory accretions.

Ayurvedic rejuvenation practices usually follow Pancha Karma or a period of internal cleansing. They are combined with Yoga and meditation, because if the mind is not renewed, the body cannot be either. They use many of the special rejuvenative herbs mentioned above. They often require a period of weeks or months in retreat in nature, as society is filled with the forces of decay. Yet if we live according to our individual nature, with the proper life-regime, that itself is productive of longevity, even if we do not resort to such specific rejuvenation practices.

4
THE SCIENCE OF LIGHT
VEDIC ASTROLOGY

Astrology has been regarded all over the world as the foremost of the occult sciences. It is the primary Vedanga or limb of the Vedas, as through it is determined the right timing of actions. It is called the science of reason or causes "Hetu Shastra" as through it we can discern the karmic patterns behind events. Another name for it is "Jyotish," the science of light, as it deals with the subtle astral light patterns which inform and sustain our physical being and determine our destiny in life. Some form of astrology was used in most ancient cultures to aid all aspects of life. In the Vedic culture as in others it set forth the ritual and the calendar and the main sacraments and initiations of life. The ancients did not look to the stars out of mental curiosity or primitive superstition but according to a profound reverence for the power of the cosmos. It was their means of making their action in harmony with the rhythms of the universe. Modern science also shows us a mysterious, dynamic and cataclysmic universe which we must pay homage to but has yet to provide us with a means of tuning into it to guide what we do.

Vedic astrology is not just another system of astrological interpretation. Its purpose is not just to tell us what our destiny is via the stars. It does not leave us helpless before fate but shows how we can use the planetary energies operative in our lives in the best possible way. It also has a practical side, its Yoga. This is its series of remedial measures aimed at purifying our subtle or psychic environment, balancing our planetary influences and maximizing our karma. Its methods include the use of gems, colors, mantras, deities, rituals, herbs and foods. Hence, a competent Vedic astrologer can provide us with tools to harmonize our entire being with the stars and align us thereby with the beneficent forces of the entire cosmos. Astrology is the basis for a total examination of our life on all levels, inner and outer, and can be used for an integral life-counseling from which an integral life-regime can be developed.

We all clean our bodies and our houses on a regular basis. Yet few of us know how to clear our psychic or mental space. We are blind to the occult influences in the world around us. Such things as the use of rituals, mantras and the science of astrology help us to do this. The foremost of these psychic influences we have to deal with is that of the planets. Just as a person who walks around blindly is bound to come to some accident or calamity, so too by our blindness to the subtle forces of the stars we undergo many difficulties in life which are unnecessary. Even wars are often caused this way, by the impurity of our collective mental environment. Vedic astrology teaches us to see these influences and gives us the means of promoting those which are beneficial and warding off those which are harmful.

The Gods we find propitiated in ancient cultures are the planets and the stars or, to be more accurate, the subtle and cosmic forces working through them. The ancient calendar, ritual, worship and daily activity were all one. This was as true among the Mayans of the New World, as the Hindus and Egyptians of the old. Each hour, day, month and year relates to a particular form of the Divine or aspect of the cosmic energy. Understanding their qualities, our actions can remain in harmony with the universe and act with its power. Even today the rituals done in India usually include the worship of the planets.

Such attitudes and actions are not based on fear or ignorance but on an understanding of the cosmic order and the interrelationship of man and the universe. The circling of the planets is not separate from the flowing of blood in our body, of impulses through our senses or thoughts through our mind. In fact, it is only through the movement of the planets that the other actions of life on Earth are possible. We live in a world of tremendous forces. It is an awesome and spectacular universe. It was the understanding of this power from which the science of astrology originated.

We pride ourselves in having gone beyond the limited views of ancient and medieval cultures. We have left the earth centered view of the solar system and look upon the ancients who saw the earth as the center of the universe to have been naive. We have broken through many other divisions of race, language and culture and find traditional cultures like India to be still caught in these narrow patterns. But we have not gone beyond what may be the most basic of all illusions and self-centered thinking processes, the materialistic idea of the world. We are almost entirely engrossed in the physical world as the sole reality and our personal ego as our real identity. While these traditional cultures had much less understanding or comprehension of the physical world than we do, they also had more knowledge of the subtle worlds and the spiritual reality behind them than we do. They would regard us as very naive and self-centered in this regard, tied to the sensory view of the world and blocked to any deeper intuition or inner perception. It is from this deeper perception they developed and used astrology. Though it may have been naive to outer realities, it does give us a better picture of the occult forces at work in life. As modern science begins to question the reality of time and space and the visible world, it may come to know these forces and appreciate more why the ancients took these more seriously than the forces of the outer world.

Modern science deals with the sensory perceivable and measurable world. Astrology deals more with the astral world than the physical, with the energy behind form rather than the forms themselves and with the energy of the mind more so than the energy of matter. It tells us that the visible is the outcome of invisible forces, that the forms of things follow impulses in the mind. As such, it is not contrary to modern science, but is a subtler form of science which can be added to it. To appreciate it we cannot just take an outer view of things. We must acknowledge our unity with all of life and discern how the forces of the cosmos, particularly those of the planets, affect us. While the effect of the Moon on life on Earth is well known, we have not examined those of the other planets with enough depth to discover their similarly significant actions.

Astrology can be validated through tests and experiments. Yet these must be sensitive to the level on which it is operating. It is not enough just to compare the Sun signs of people. What is necessary is to study many charts on an individual basis, noting not only how the same specific planetary factors may occur in each but also how overall patterns relate. To study the occurrence of a disease in the human body we have to note many patterns and combinations of external and internal factors. It does not follow a few simplistic interpretations. Astrology must be approached with the same comprehensiveness and intricacy of approach as any science. If we do this, we find a profound connection between the birth chart and the nature of our lives and characters. We find many connections between the charts of those of similar destinies. What remains an art in astrology is the spiritual interpretation of the chart, as this transcends outer factors.

Classical Vedic astrology uses the seven visible planets: the Sun, Moon, Mars, Mercury, Jupiter, Venus and Saturn, along with the two lunar nodes, the north and south nodes, Rahu and Ketu. Some modern practitioners incorporate Uranus, Neptune and Pluto but this is not necessary for an accurate reading. The effects of the distant planets is not as crucial. Many of their effects can be discerned through the functioning of the lunar nodes. Yet, though Vedic astrology uses fewer planets it requires more calculations than a regular western astrological chart, as it goes into much more detail in regard to the location and strength of the planets.

Vedic astrology uses the twelve signs and twelve houses and planetary aspects, much like western astrology but with some differences, particularly in regard to the aspects.

SIDEREAL ASTROLOGY

Vedic Astrology is "sidereal" in nature; that is, it is based upon the actual observable constellations for its delineations of the signs of the zodiac. Most Western astrology is "tropical" in nature. It does not use the actual fixed stars but bases its signs upon the point of the equinox, which is slowly but constantly changing in the heavens. It should be noted that there is a Western form of sidereal astrology and that Edgar Cayce often recommended this approach. Tibetan astrology is also based upon the Vedic sidereal model.

Owing to the precession of the equinoxes, the point of the vernal equinox is now in early Pisces moving towards Aquarius; hence, the idea that the age of Aquarius now dawning. In normal Western astrology the point of the vernal equinox is always considered to be the first point of Aries, regardless of its actual point in the heavens. By Aries it is not referring to the stars of the constellation Aries. It is a symbol or abstraction that can be applied to any section of the stars of the zodiac which serves to mark the vernal equinox.

If we look at a regular ephemeris and see that the Moon is in Gemini and then go out and see what constellation it is actually in, we will most likely find it in the stars of Taurus, which is where Vedic astrology would place it. Hence, sidereal astrology is more astronomically accurate and reflects more the stars. Tropical astrology reflects more the seasonal changes and the Sun-Earth relationship. Both systems have their efficacy but their languages may confuse us, as what they refer to as the signs of the zodiac is determined by two different standards of measurement. It is not in doubt where the signs actually are, but the method of ascertaining them has two main methods which yield different results.

Sidereal astrology calculates this ongoing movement of the precession into its planeary positions. Hence, its point for the vernal equinox is slowly changing, a rate around 50″ per year.

According to the standard government of India system, the equinox will be as of 1990 about 6° 20′ of Pisces. In the Puranas, the mythological texts of late ancient and medieval India, we read of the spring equinox as at 0° Aries (c. 500 A.D.). In *Vedanga Jyotish,* a late Vedic supplement, we find it in the end of Aries (c. 1200 B.C.). In most later Vedic texts we find it in the Pleiades or early Taurus (c. 2000 B.C.). In earlier Vedic mythology we find it near the beginning of Gemini or Orion (c. 4000 B.C.), or at the beginning of Cancer (c. 6000 B.C.), with yet earlier references all the way back to Libra (c. 12,000 B.C.). The astrologers of India kept track of the shifting of the equinoxes. As the calendar was based upon the position of the equinox to determine the months, many changes of calendar similar to our age of Aquarius are found instituted in different parts of the Vedic teachings. Unlike Europe in the Middle Ages, the astrologers in India, many of whom were yogis, never forgot the fact of the precession. For this reason, in sidereal astrology our zodiacal sign placements will usually change. They will generally fall back one sign. The Sun signs in sidereal astrology usually change around the 14th of the month. Hence, Aries is April 14-May 14; Taurus, May 14-June 14; Gemini, June 14-July 14; Cancer, July 14-August 14; Leo, Aug.14-Sept.14; Virgo, Sept.14-Oct.14; Libra, Oct.14-Nov.14; Scorpio, Nov.14-Dec.14; Sagittarius, Dec.14-Jan.14; Capricorn, Jan.14-Feb.14; Aquarius, Feb.14-March 14; and Pisces, March 14-April 14. As there is not an exact agreement among all sidereal astrologers as to the degree and rate of the precession, the date may vary by a day or two either way depending upon the system used.

Sidereal astrology holds that there is a constant connection between certain stars and certain sections of the sky and life on Earth. It is based on the galactic center which marks the beginning of Sagittarius, the positive sign of Jupiter, the planet called in Sanskrit "guru," the Divine teacher. Jupiter brings into our solar system the beneficent influences from the galactic center. Presently, the winter solstice is now in conjunction with the galactic center. It will be exact around 2100 A.D. As such, we are witnessing a new influx of spiritual energy from that galactic sun.

Another important point of orientation for the zodiac is the star Vega. It marked the north pole around 12,000 B.C. In the Vedic system this is said to be the main star governing the movement of our Sun, its local ruler.

In the cycles of the World-ages (yugas) used in Vedic astrology, we are now said to have recently entered the second age (Dwapara Yuga), called the Bronze age by the Greeks. It is an era of rapid development of scientific knowledge, leading gradually into the occult. It is destined to last another two thousand years, as part of a 24,000 year cycle. Yet we are still in a longer age of Kali Yuga or the Iron Age lasting 432,000 years, making the mentality of the majority of human beings still tending towards materialism even in the ages of light of the shorter cycle. Nevertheless, we all have the power to transcend our destiny, as our inner soul is inherently free of karma. It is not the stars which bind us, but our attachment to the external world which, in turn, places us under the rule of its forces.

PLANETARY TYPES

Vedic astrology judges individuals not so much by their Sun or any other sign but according to their predominant planet. Usually, it considers the Ascendant or rising sign to be the most important factor, then the Moon and third the Sun. The Ascendant represents the physical body and material incarnation; the Moon the mind and emotional nature; the Sun the self or soul and rationality. The predominant planet is usually that which most influences the Ascendant, Moon, Sun or their lords.

Solar Types

Solar types have a moderate build, a glowing or golden complexion and appear to give light, particularly through their eyes. They have strong hearts, good circulation and strong vitality. They are dignified, command respect, make good leaders, have a fatherly disposition and are noble and strong. They have a good sense of truth, right, order, law and justice. They seek power, status, preeminence and prestige and like to be leaders. They have good wills and strong characters but can be vain, proud, critical or opinionated. They are often dramatic and like to be the center of attention. They like to shine on all the world and to have all the world look to them for light and warmth.

Lunar Types

Lunar types have round features, usually white complexion and tend towards obesity or water retention. They have a certain luminosity about them. They are friendly, sociable, open, caring, non-violent, concerned with the welfare of others and often possess a maternal disposition. They treat others as members of their own family. They can be shy and sensitive, passive, withdrawn or fearful and may be dominated by their moods, sentiments or emotions. Yet when more evolved, they can become leaders, administrators and very diplomatic. They can be popular and know how to influence the masses. They also like to shine and like others to find happiness or delight in their company.

Mars Types

Mars types usually possess a ruddy complexion, with some angularity or sharpness in their features. They may have scars, wounds, or get injured easily. They are usually well built and have good muscle tone but have hot blood and tend towards febrile and infectious diseases. They are bold, daring, aggressive, perhaps contentious and may get into conflicts. They like discipline, are militaristic and easily form alliances. They are strong workers, rational and practically minded, and are often technically or scientifically oriented and can do much with their hands. They like action, energy and the display of force.

Mercury Types

Mercury types are intelligent, communicative, good at speech, witty, quick with information and ideas. They tend to be nervous, sensitive, agitated, and fast in their movements. They make good writers, secretaries, businessmen, teachers, and administrators. They are very adaptable and flexible in their attitudes and manner and can be diplomatic and humane. Physically they are also agile, flexible and fast but may lack in endurance. They are often humorous and good at imitating others. They are easily influenced and find it hard to hold to any decisions.

Jupiter Types

Jupiter types are expansive, happy, optimistic and accomplish a great deal in life. They are usually large or well built, stocky with a strong constitution, good health and longevity. They are physically, mentally and socially active and like to do things with others. They are intelligent, philosophical or religious in nature, though not always good at details. They have good faith and compassion, yet they can be too orthodox or opinionated, trapped in the religious or political patterns of their given culture. They can overextend themselves, and may accumulate too much in life. Fortune and grace usually go with them but can take them too far.

Venus Types

Venus types are attractive, well-proportioned, charming, good-looking and graceful. They often have a strong sexual energy and beautiful faces, with a certain feminine quality about them. They are artistic and creative and like beauty, comfort or luxury. While they can have a good deal of love and devotion, they may dissipate themselves with sensuality and become trapped in glamor and seduction. They possess good imaginations, a strong sense of color and have vivid dreams. When more evolved they easily gain occult knowledge or perception or the power of devotion.

Saturn Types

Saturn types tend to be gaunt, lean, with dry skin, darkness around the eyes and irregular features. They may have large noses, large or crooked teeth, or unattractive features. They are often coarse, unfeeling or perhaps rough in nature. They may come from the lower strata of society or be outside of social recognition. They are solitary, serious, or depressed. They are difficult to relate to and seldom have many friends. They often suffer in life, have bad luck, poverty or disease. When they are successful, it takes time, effort and struggle, and they may be selfish and conservative in what they gain. When unevolved, they may be selfish and cold. When highly evolved they are detached and calm, philosophical and meditative.

Rahu (North Node) Types

Rahu types are mysterious, unpredictable, dark and elusive, some-times ghostly. They are easily excited and carried away by influences and are creatures of fantasy and astral forces. They can be easily disturbed and are often afflicted in mind and body with mysterious diseases, mental or nervous system disorders. They often have weak immune systems or allergies. They often have many unrealistic projections in life, but others also easily make unrealistic projections upon them.

Ketu (South Node) Types

Ketu types are critical, sharp in perception but narrow in perspective and often tied to a narrow or archaic point of view. They possess much insight but sometimes little comprehension. They can possess great mastery over what they set their will upon. They are eccentric, individu-alistic and sometimes arouse the anger of others. They are susceptible to contagious disease or to mass calamities. When highly evolved they gain the highest spiritual knowledge as they learn how to negate all things into the sole reality of the inner Self.

SHADBALA
Means of Determining Planetary Strengths

Shadbala is an elaborate means of determining the strength and weakness of planets. It require extensive calculation but can be easily done by computer programs. It mainly shows how strong planets are in terms of location and temporal factors. It considers a whole range of conditions including the position of the planets in the birth and harmonic charts, the phases of the Moon, seasons of the year, times of the day, the motion of the planets and planetary aspects.

HARMONIC CHARTS

Vedic astrology employs up to sixteen harmonic charts (including the basic birth chart). These are based upon subdivisions of the birth chart and allow us to give a more fine-tuned meaning to the affairs of life. Aspects, signs and houses can also come from these charts. Western astrology is just beginning to employ such subtle charts. Most important is the ninth harmonic (navamsha), as this shows the inner meaning of the life and the nature of the soul.

PLANETARY SIGNIFICATORS
(Karakas)

Planets signify different aspects of our nature. This is based upon how many degrees they are in any particular sign. The planet with the highest number of degrees becomes the significator of the Self (Atmakaraka) and tells much about our inner nature and spiritual evolution. Its position in the harmonic ninth and other subtle charts is very important for showing this.

PLANETARY PERIODS
(Dashas and Bhuktis)

Vedic astrology employs a special system of planetary periods. In these each planet rules a period of time in life from six to twenty years. The main cycle used (Vimshottari Dasha), one hundred and twenty years, is as follows:

The Sun	Six years
The Moon	Ten years
Mars	Seven years
Rahu	Eighteen years
Jupiter	Sixteen years
Saturn	Nineteen years
Mercury	Seventeen years
Venus	Twenty years
Ketu	Seven years

Each of these major periods (Dashas) is divided into minor periods (Bhuktis) based upon the same proportions per planet.

Where the cycle begins depends upon the location of the Moon at birth.

The planetary periods are very important for determining the courses of events in life. All of us would benefit from knowing their periods. If this is all we take from Vedic astrology it is well worth it. It should be noted that transits are also considered but relative to these more general periods.

REMEDIAL MEASURES
Gem Therapy

To each of the planets is prescribed a particular gemstone.

These are:

The Sun	Ruby
The Moon	Pearl
Mars	Red Coral
Mercury	Emerald
Jupiter	Yellow Sapphire
Venus	Diamond
Saturn	Blue Sapphire
Rahu	Hessonite Garnet
Ketu	Cat's Eye (Chrysoberyl)

Gemstones are usually prescribed when a planet is weak in the chart (by sign, house, or aspect) and particularly if it also rules auspicious houses from the ascendant (like the first, fifth or ninth).

Ruby and yellow sapphire are usually set in gold. Pearl and red coral are usually set in silver. Diamond is set in white gold (a combination of gold and silver). Emerald, and blue sapphire can be set in either gold or silver depending on whether we want to strengthen their cleansing or nourishing effects.

The gemstones follow the color of the rays transmitted by the planets. Substitute gems are garnet or sunstone for the ruby; moonstone or cloudy quartz crystal for pearl; red carnelian for red coral; peridot, jade or green tourmaline for emerald; yellow topaz, yellow zircon or citrine for yellow sapphire; amethyst, lapis or dark blue turquoise for blue sapphire; clear zircon or clear quartz crystal for diamond; golden grossularite garnet for hessonite; other forms of cat's eye for chrysoberyl cat's eye.

Gemstones are usually worn on the fingers ruled by the planet or one of its friendly planets. The index finger is ruled by Jupiter and also can take gems for Mars, the Sun or the Moon. The middle finger is ruled by Saturn and also can take gems for Mercury or Venus. The ring finger is ruled by the Sun but also can take gems for the Moon, Mars and Jupiter. The little finger is ruled by Mercury but can also take gems for Venus. Rahu can be treated like Saturn and Ketu like Mars.

Gemstones should be good quality, without flaws, preferably a minimum of three carats in size and set so as to touch the skin. It is best to put them on during days, hours or periods favorable to the planet they relate to.

Vedic astrology holds that all gems are like transmitters. They bring in the energy of a particular planet. But it is up to us on what level we use that energy. Strengthening Mercury, for example, may give the powers of the lower or the higher mind. Hence, mantras, meditation and the power of our intentions are needed along with the gems to insure their higher or more spiritual affect.

Planets and Deities

Each planet relates to a particular deity. While there are several versions of this system, I prefer that given below.

The Sun	The Great God or Divine Father, Shiva.
The Moon	The Great Goddess or Divine Mother, Parvati.
Mars	Skanda, the war God, son of Shiva.
Mercury	Vishnu, the Divine Preserver.
Jupiter	Brihaspati, the priest of the Gods (by other accounts Ganesh, the elephant God).
Venus	Lakshmi, the Goddess of Beauty.
Saturn	The dark or old forms of the God and Goddess, Shiva and Kali.
Rahu	Durga, the terrible and protective form of the Goddess.
Ketu	Rudra, the terrible and protective form of the God, Shiva.

We can take our preferred or chosen deity (whatever it may be) and use it to ward off the negative effects of planetary influences also. The nature of the deity does not matter as much as the energy of devotion that we direct towards it.

VEDIC AND WESTERN ASTROLOGY

Vedic astrology represents the oldest, most consistent and most continually used system of astrology in the world. It was established and handed down through a series of enlightened sages including by many great yogis up to the present. Shri Yukteswar, guru of Paramahansa Yogananda, was one such great yogic astrologer.

Additionally, as it corresponds to the fixed stars, it cannot be criticized by astronomers for no longer being accurate, as is the case with tropical astrology. It is more scientific and based more clearly on direct observation.

Vedic astrology involves a shift in the sign positions in the chart, which makes it hard to understand for those used to their tropical positions. Two-thirds of us will find our Sun signs changing, as well as the signs of all our other planets. If we are already used to reading ourselves by the standards of tropical astrology this shift may prove difficult to deal with. We might find it hard to change from being a Virgo to a Leo Sun, for example.

It should be noted that neither system, the sidereal or the tropical is wrong. They just base their measurement of the signs on different factors. Ancient astrology, however, all over the world, was sidereal in nature because it was originally based on direct observation. The ancients could not have employed a symbolic tropical zodiac. When they said the Moon in Taurus, it had to be observable among the stars there.

Unfortunately, the language of Vedic Astrology is still largely medieval, like that of older western astrology and its moralistic pronouncements. It is tied to older Indian cultural patterns which are no longer relevant in the modern world. Many classical or traditional texts are for this reason very hard for westerners to understand. Even some easterners prefer books on western astrology over their own for reason of their broader social concepts. However, a modern form of Vedic astrology is arising that is free of this complication.

Vedic astrology can also be used along with or to supplement Western astrology either in its tropical or sidereal forms. Indeed, many aspects of Vedic astrology are already being introduced into Western astrology, like the harmonic charts.

Some say Vedic or Hindu astrology applies for Hindus and Western astrology for westerners. This is another form of cultural prejudice which inhibits objectivity. While both systems have some cultural limitations, we should note that the stars and planets should not be held to operate according to them. Vedic astrology can be used to give quite accurate readings for westerners and Western astrology can work very good on Hindus.

There are those who say that Vedic astrology is good for prediction but Western astrology has a better psychological and spiritual usage. This is because many Hindu astrologers, living in a fixed and traditional culture, tend to use astrology just to predict or order the outer affairs of life, when and to whom someone will marry, what kind of work they will do, without any consideration of the psychological issues that may be involved. We see the same thing in medieval western astrology. However, this does not faithfully represent Vedic science or the many great Yogis who have used this system. Vedic astrology is quite useful for pointing out our spiritual path in life and giving us a means to connect with the Divine via our planetary forces. It is true it is not so much concerned with outer psychology, our personal and emotional issues. But it is concerned with inner psychology, the spiritual purpose of our life. In this regard it is much more developed than Western astrology, which but for a few exceptions does not even recognize liberation or self-realization as the ultimate goal of life or understand the patterns of karma and rebirth. An entire aspect of Vedic astrology is considered with our potential for liberation in life.

Vedic astrology may, therefore, also be the astrology of the future. Certainly, it will only be after many years of comparative usage of sidereal and tropical systems that their respective validity will emerge along with the forms of them which are likely to endure. Yet astrology will always remain with us, as it is as constant as our connection with the stars.

5
VEDIC SOCIAL SCIENCE
THE SPIRITUAL BASIS OF CULTURE

THE BACKGROUND OF SOCIETY

All societies possess a certain structure. At certain times in all cultures various leaders arise who establish the social order, which then is followed until the next great change or renovation. Such leaders are the great founders of our cultures, and each culture has those whom it honors. They establish eras in history, and time periods are often based upon them. It is the values that they establish which determine how the particular culture develops.

When we examine human beings from the standpoint of society we find that different people have different aptitudes and come in different types. We have different values and attitudes and do not all want the same thing. Divisions are by age, sex, race, religion, occupation and so on. It is hard enough to understand ourselves in one to one individual interaction. To create an understanding between the diverse groups within humanity appears almost impossible. Hence, for any society to exist a certain amount of tolerance and accommodation of differing views is required. Moreover, a certain objective structure is required which all these different groups can recognize, with definite laws or values and some means of enforcing them. The mindsets of individuals are so variable that without some objective standard any long term social cohesion cannot be maintained.

The ancients, perhaps surprising to us, were more conscious about their social structures than we are. They had smaller groups of people and could more easily establish defined cultural orders. They designed their social orders in a particular way that seems rigid to us today. They kept a stricter control of marriage and social intercourse. They had clear and often rigid distinctions of roles and classes, as well as a sharp division of the sexes.

Modern societies have usually been restructured after some great political event, a revolution or a reform like the American revolution, and thereby have a primarily secular order. Ancient societies were based upon religious renovations; the code of Moses or Mohammed. The law giver was often the prophet or sage or aligned with him. The social order was not established by man at some point of history, as is the case with modern societies, but brought down from God, from a connection with the eternal. While such religious cultures may appear superstitious to us or based on wishful thinking, they certainly have been able to endure longer than our secular ones. No secular culture has yet to stand the test of time. Hence, we may be wise to reexamine the meaning of culture from the standpoint of religion and spirituality.

In the primitive state of humanity, the pretechnological and pre-civilization stage, each individual or family had to fulfill the different actions necessary for the maintenance of life. They had to function for providing their own food, clothing, shelter, protection, education and religious guidance. In the course of time a natural diversification of roles occurred. By concentrating on one action more could be accomplished. One man became a farmer, the other built houses, the third taught the lore of the people, and so on. By a greater expertise in these different roles society could provide a richer life for all. However, in this process independence and self-reliance became reduced. The individual became progressively more dependent upon society and its definitions to fulfill his basic necessities. Conflict arose as to the relative value or importance of each role. Generally, the manual roles were considered inferior to those occupations done with the mind, like the role of the priest. The roles which dealt with the broader life of the people, social or religious, gained more prestige than those limited to the needs of the person or family. For example, the head of the community was regarded as more important than the common laborer.

THE CLASS STRUCTURE

All ancient and medieval cultures up to the past few centuries in the West and many of those still existing elsewhere in the world have been based upon the same general idea. This is the division of society into several major groups according to an organic differentiation of functions.

These are the classes of the priests, nobility, and the common people; the latter usually divided into merchants and farmers. Within this are usually other subcastes like artists and craftsmen. This idea which we still find in its petrified form in the caste system of India was the universal idea of the ancient mind. It appeared to the ancient mind to represent the natural order, to be self-evident. We find it among the Mayans, Aztecs and Incas of the New World. We see it in ancient Egypt, Babylonia, Assyria, Persia, as well as India and China. Even Christian Europe in the Middle Ages followed it.

While we may want to dismiss it today as a form of social inequality and political oppression, it is not wise simply to reject ideas according to the forms they may have degenerated into in time. If this idea was so universal, it had a meaning and a purpose, it reflected a certain truth that must have had some validity at least for a time.

Such social orders reflect a different idea of the world and a more intimate connection with nature. We could call them organic, whereas our democratic or communist social orders are conceptual. All human beings may not simply be equal in terms of their function, any more than the organs of the body are. The brain has one function and the stomach has another. We cannot give half of the work of the brain to the stomach or half of the work of the stomach to the brain. Such equality would kill us. Nor should the stomach be allowed to function as the brain. A right organic order may be essential to society. It should not be confused with a conceptual order or with a wrong organic order (such as most of these older cultures degenerated into).

We should also note that these cultural orders were far less rigid at their origin. While a difference in function was acknowledged, each role was regarded as necessary and sacred. Only in time was the organic social order divided into rigid compartments rather than complementary functions. The farmer was not originally inferior to the king. Both were seen as providing essential functions. Though one may have been subordinate to the other, each had its important place in the sacred order. Hence, it was the king who did the first plowing for the year.

Even in our modern culture these same different types have their own different, though not as isolated, social orders. The priests or religious people of any group tend to form their own community, as with monasteries and churches. The nobility, our political leaders, also have their own echelon of society, which requires a certain background to be able to enter. The army has its own territory and laws and is a society within society. While we may have eliminated the formality of slavery, we still have our servant and poverty classes, along with their ghettos. Such divisions tend to occur according to the different attitudes and aptitudes of people, and they can breed conflict and suspicion whether they are formalized or not. They can be used by one group of society to control or take advantage of the others.

There is, therefore, a natural tendency or need to form different subcultures within society. While it certainly can become a form of oppression, it may have an appropriate form we have to adjust to. Such diversification may be necessary for the full flowering of the different potentials of humanity or for the development of the full range of experience necessary for the human soul to grow. We are not all of one level in humanity. We do not all have the same goals in life. Souls are not all of the same stage of development. Just as there are different classes in a school that appeal to students of different temperaments, like science, mathematics or art, so there may need to be different areas of learning in society for different souls to pursue. Some may need to pursue business as an exclusive aim, others politics, others knowledge or art. Just as there are different grades in school, so grades in society may also exist. There may be a spiritual class which has advanced beyond ordinary humanity to the point where we should look up to it for guidance.

THE VEDIC SOCIAL ORDER

The ancient culture of India was based upon such a system of social diversification according to spiritual development. It was consciously formed along those lines many thousands of years ago. Though we see it only in the distance today, we can still ascertain its relevance if we examine it deeply. It may again become a model for the future.

The founder of this ancient Hindu or Aryan society, the culture of spiritual humanity, was called Manu, from whose name the term man arises. He is the Vedic Noah, the great leader who survived the mythical flood and established the new social order, reflecting a return to spiritual values from an earlier and materialistic humanity that had fallen from its spiritual foundation, which somewhat like our society today, had violated the laws of God and Nature and thereby brought down its own destruction.

Manu recognized four orders of society based upon the four main goals of human beings and established society accordingly. These four groups were the Brahmins, the priests or spiritual class; the Kshatriya, the nobility or ruling class; the Vaishya, the merchants and farmers; and the Shudras or servants.

In the *Rig Veda*, the oldest scripture of India, three basic classes are noted; the Brahmin, the Kshatriya or Rajanya, and the Vish, which latter means literally the people. Hence, there was one basic class of humanity with two orders to guide it, a spiritual order or the Brahmins and a political order or the Kshatriya.

These four orders of society were called varna, which has two meanings; first it means color and second it means a veil. As color it does not refer to the color of the skin of people, as some superficially minded scholars have believed, but to the qualities or energies of human nature. As a veil it shows the four different ways in which the Divine Self is hidden in human beings.

The four energies of human beings are the white, red, yellow and black. White is the quality of sattva; of purity, clarity, love, faith and detachment. It prevails in those of spiritual temperament; those seeking true knowledge, who alone deserve the name of Brahmin. Red is the quality of rajas; of action, will, aggression, energy, its impulse towards achievement. It prevails in those of martial and political temperament; those seeking honor, fame, status and power. It is these who are the Kshatriyas. Yellow is another quality of rajas, its impulse towards accumulation, towards communication, interchange, trade, business. It prevails in those of commercial temperament, the Vaishyas. Black is the color of tamas, of darkness, ignorance, inertia and dullness. It prevails in those of servile disposition, those dependent on the external world for their motivation. These are the true Shudras.

These four energies are the four main powers of Nature in human beings. They are the movements of the cosmic Nature (Prakriti) in man. They are the four main ways of action for all human beings of all times and places. What determines them is not some social custom or convenience but the attributes of our nature. This is revealed by our values in life, by what we really believe in our hearts. It can be ascertained by what we spend the greatest amount of our time pursuing. If we are mainly occupied in pursuing spiritual knowledge, we are a Brahmin. If we are mainly concerned with accumulating money, we belong to the commercial class. If we are mainly after pleasure we are of the servile class.

Birth and family can be an important factor in determining this but, in itself, it is not enough to indicate it. We sometimes see people of spiritual disposition born in commercial families. We sometimes see people of commercial disposition born in a line of priests.

The man of spiritual knowledge understands all these four orders of society and is capable of functioning in any of them. He sees them as different aspects of his own nature; the laborers as his legs, the merchants as his belly, the nobility as his arms and the priests as his head. Until we reach this perspective, we cannot go beyond rebirth in the human world.

As long as the social order in ancient India was maintained and the dharma or religious practice of the family continued, birth could be relied on most of the time as the indication of an individual's place in the social order. But according to the *Bhagavad Gita,* this Aryan family system broke down in India over three thousand years ago at the time of Krishna. Hence, after three thousand years this system of determining natural aptitude has degenerated into the caste system which resembles it now only in form.

THE STRUCTURE OF HUMAN SOCIETY

There are only a few basic values or goals in life we can pursue. This is owing to the limited nature of our lives, our body, senses and mind. While we may think there is any number of things we can pursue, they resolve themselves into a few areas: pleasure, wealth, power and knowledge.

The most basic goal is pleasure, to enjoy ourselves in life, primarily enjoyment of the senses (kama). While a certain amount of pleasure in our natural functioning is necessary for harmonious action in life, we usually seek it far beyond this.

The second goal is wealth, which is the accumulation of the necessary objects to provide for our well-being (artha). The most basic are food, clothing and shelter, but beyond these we seek objects to make our lives more comfortable or convenient or simply more ostentatious.

The third goal is power or status, which is the achievement of a certain recognition or fame for ourselves (dharma). For us to accomplish anything in life we have to have a certain status or reputation. Without that no one knows who we are or what we can do. Yet beyond this natural need we seek to have power over others and to exalt ourselves at the expense of others.

The fourth goal is freedom (moksha), which is our ability to transcend the outer world and our limited place within it. The external world is produced by time and is subject to death. We all seek something eternal or lasting so that our life has some enduring meaning. Freedom depends upon knowledge. Hence, this is also the goal of knowledge Through knowledge we can extend ourselves beyond the limits of our bodies and senses and thereby attain things which even wealth and power cannot provide.

Knowledge, however, is higher or lower. The lower knowledge, that of the intellect, gives us mastery of the outer world. It is only the higher knowledge or self-knowledge which provides for the liberation of the spirit or the true goal of life. How a society defines what is true knowledge is the indication of its ultimate goal and value.

These four goals produce four classes or strata of human beings. We can call these the laborers or working class, the merchants or commercial class, the political and military class, and the intellectual and spiritual class. We still have them today and, while they are not official castes, there are definite barriers between them which are hard to cross over.

In ancient cultures all these roles were tied with some religious or spiritual purpose. Now they are purely of a secular or profane nature. In the religious orders of the ancient world the laborers worked for the spiritual good of the society by providing not only food for themselves but also for the priests and the monks. The merchants set aside a certain portion of their wealth to provide for both the lower and the higher classes, to give shelter to the poor or to build churches and temples. The warriors served to protect the whole society from invasions which would disrupt it. The priests dispensed knowledge to all and kept the society in harmony with the cosmic order.

Actually, all the outer values of life tend to go together. They are all based on an external seeking and keep us dependent upon external influences. Pleasure, wealth, power and outer knowledge are all based upon desire. We seek wealth and power to give us more pleasure. We seek knowledge to give us more wealth and power. Only spiritual knowledge is an inner value.

Our values determine our life experience. They color our perception and determine our view of the world. The merchant sees the world in terms of money or saleable goods. His perception of the world is bound by commercial values. The political person sees it in terms of political power, national identity, party affiliation, etc. The religious person sees it according to his belief and judges people by theirs. A subclass like the artist sees it in his way, according to his aesthetic values.

If our primary goal in life is pleasure we develop a servile attitude in life. The pursuit of pleasure is the pursuit of the external, coming under the influence or domination of the senses, which places us under the control of our environment and its sources of pleasure and pain, reward and punishment. We pursue immediate sensation and gratification, which in turn deprives us of a life plan or purpose through which we could master our destiny.

If our primary goal in life is wealth, we develop a commercial attitude. We see things in terms of how much money we can make through them or how much property we can accumulate by them. This also causes us to manipulate the world and other people to gain more for ourselves.

If our primary goal in life is power or status, then we develop ambition. We want to become somebody, gain recognition, become famous. We create followers for ourselves and subordinate others to our drives.

If our goal in life is knowledge then we develop the intellect. We seek pleasure, acquisition and achievement through the mind rather than through the body, senses or outer world. Through our accumulation of ideas we gain control of others.

There are no other possible outer goals for us in life than these. We may change their forms, but their basic nature must remain the same. We may develop new and more exciting forms of pleasure but the experience of pleasure is essentially the same. It can be a little more or less, but it cannot become qualitatively different. To gain the same experience of pleasure, however, we need ever new objects or more powerful forms, as what is stimulating the first time becomes less exciting through repetition.

These goals are all outward, limited and transient. They are bound by death. Whatever we gain of them in life cannot become a permanent part of our being or improve our state of awareness. They cannot provide any lasting happiness, abundance, energy or wisdom.

We still pursue these goals all over the world. We have expanded their fields horizontally, but we remain under their rule. Through the pursuit of pleasure we can only gain pleasure. The senses themselves are limited and can easily be damaged or exhausted by pushing pleasure beyond its limited scope. While a new stereo may appear to give more pleasure than an old one, the simple experience of the sound of a bird heard by an innocent mind is far greater than any of these. Our expanded field may only complicate, not improve, our condition.

Through the pursuit of wealth we can only gain wealth. It will gives us bigger houses, better cars, more jewels, but will not give us true happiness or immortality. A simple man may gain the same feeling through finding a beautiful rock on a hill, as a wealthy man through earning his latest million.

Through the pursuit of status we can only gain status. This gives us fame, recognition and adulation. But it cannot provide peace, integrity, and a true sense of self-worth. The recognition by society of our being a famous person may be less genuine than the recognition by our wife or partner of our integrity in life.

Though the forms of these values can change, their basic nature remains the same, and the type of life we can experience from them is of the same order. For example, the life of a merchant in ancient Egypt and one in the United States today does differ greatly in form, but the basic mentality and emotions are going to be the same. Hence, as long as we pursue these same values, we are only expanding our society horizontally. We are not actually bringing in any ascent or spiritual evolution.

Our values in life serve to divide us. When they come into conflict we find ourselves at odds with each other. As long as we are pursuing lower values or personal gains, such strife is inevitable. If my values are commercial, I must come into conflict with the commercial needs of others as wealth is always limited. Society can only be truly united through religious or spiritual values which transcend human differences and limited resources.

THE LIMITATIONS OF DEMOCRACY

The ancients did not believe in a simple democracy or equality between men. They saw an equality between the souls of men but realized that our human aptitudes are quite different, our minds and their values differ. There is in democracy, its negative side, the scaling down of higher values, just as there is in it the raising up of the lower classes. It aims at the average, which may be the mediocre.

It also serves to impose one set of values upon all human beings. These are defined by the values behind the democracy. In most democracies they are economic freedom or commercial interests. Hence, they naturally impose commercial values on the whole of society. They do not just simply allow individuals to pursue different values but overtly or covertly promote the values of one level of society, the business class. This is not so much a society free of class as a society ruled by, defined by and reduced to, one class. Compared to such a one-dimensional or linear society, the ancient cultures were intricate and multidimensional.

While democracy may be better than a false hierarchy, it remains inferior to a hierarchy of real values. It can only be an intermediate phase between the degenerate ancient hierarchy and a revised futuristic one. Society cannot be free of hierarchy. Each society has its standards and authorities. We can either base it on a true set of values defined by a spiritual evolution or it will establish itself according to the lower values of wealth, power and pleasure.

The outer goals of life have their necessity, but it is only superficial. They are not the real aim. Our purpose in incarnation is to grow in consciousness. For our functioning we need certain objects to allow us to live. We need to have a certain pleasure in what we do. We need to be recognized for our skills so that we can contribute to society. We need some knowledge about the outer world. This is like a man on a journey spending a few days to gather experience in a different land. He needs to be able to provide for himself during his stay. But his real home is elsewhere. He cannot lose sight of the fact that he is only a traveler, in transit. He must pursue his primary goal, which is to return home.

We see, therefore, that the Vedic system of social science of Manu is universal. It is a conscious organization of the different aptitudes of humanity. It applies in all cultures. We must belong to one of the four varnas. The variation in culture is according to which of the varnas is given power or priority. Though we may have advanced in terms of outer power and knowledge, we have created a society that does not even recognize the validity of the spiritual goal at all. We acknowledge religion but not the true goal of the liberation of the Spirit as the real end of man. Hence, our social order is spiritually naive and bound to create some calamity for itself in time by its lack of recognition of the real purpose of life.

Until, following the principles of Manu or the true man, we return to a society whose pillar is the respect for spiritual and self-knowledge, our world must be beset with conflict and contradiction and few will be able to arrive at any real or lasting happiness.

The higher man, however, is one who realizes his unity with all humanity, one who understands the values and needs of all the levels of society. He helps each individual to pursue their appropriate path in life and does not attempt to create a single standard for all. He provides a wide field of experience in which each can grow in his own way. Such were the ancient leaders of Vedic or Aryan society.

THE FOUR STAGES OF LIFE

Besides the division of the four social orders (varna) was the Vedic division of the four stages of life (ashramas). Just as we differ in aptitudes, so do we differ in age. There are different seasons in human life as in nature. What grows in the spring will not grow in the autumn. The action that is appropriate in the spring is out of place in the fall.

In this way the normal human life was regarded as eighty-four years, consisting of four sections of twenty-one years each. The first twenty-one years is called the Brahmacharya ashram, the stage of youth or learning, which requires a certain discipline, guidance and purity for its full flowering.

The second twenty-one years, from ages twenty-one to forty-two, is called the Grihastha ashram or householder phase. This is the main time for having children and raising a family, as well as for working and fulfilling our duties to society.

The third section of twenty-one years, from ages forty-two to sixty-three is the Vanaprastha or the hermitage phase. This is a time for return to contemplation and for guiding society in the distance.

The fourth and last section from sixty-three to eighty-four is the Sannyasa or renunciation phase. The person, now an elder full of wisdom, inwardly aims to renounce all the outer goals of life. He also becomes a teacher of the spiritual knowledge and no longer partakes in social or political concerns. This order reflects the general rule. More advanced souls may go directly to the renunciation phase. Less advanced souls may not even qualify for the first phase. They may never develop the purity, innocence and humility of the Brahmacharya phase.

In this we see that only twenty-one years are allotted for the outer duties of life. Three-quarters of life is to be devoted primarily to spiritual study.

A true society provides the appropriate experiences for each of these four stages of life. Our present society is based mainly on adolescent values. Even the elderly are expected to act like the young, pursuing sex, sports and money. Such a culture is one-sided and imbalanced. The potentials of the soul in old age are denied. The natural movement of the soul in its later years towards detachment and meditation is suppressed. As the elderly naturally begin to lose interest in the outer goals of life we tell them that they are sick and encourage them to do things to remain in the mainstream of worldly seeking. The elderly are not able to grow in wisdom and become our true elders and teachers. We make them into mockeries of the young. We do not respect them and they feel we have abandoned them. As we live longer and the average age of individuals in our cultures increases, this problem becomes more acute.

Any society which does not recognize the stages of life cannot flourish for long, just as a farmer cannot be successful if he only knows the plants that flourish in one season. Nor can any individual be happy if they are following the needs of a stage of life which is no longer appropriate for them. Hence, this ancient Vedic understanding of the stages of life must be brought back again.

Society is not a two dimensional drawing. It has the invisible dimension of spiritual growth. Without recognizing this we have a warped perspective on our existence. Vedic values aid us in restoring this inner dimension to society as well as to our individual existence. It is that power of aspiration which gives true meaning to human life and allows us to appreciate the different levels and stages of our existence.

6
SANSKRIT
THE POWER OF MANTRA

Sanskrit is the language of the Vedas. It originates from the rishis, seers of the Vedas, who were said to have first envisioned it through the power of the Divine Word. The Sanskrit language is said to put forth into human sounds, the language of the Gods, the great creative cosmic vibration. It manifests from the Divine word Om, which contains within itself all sounds.

All the primary roots and forms of the Sanskrit language are present in the *Rig Veda*, the oldest of the Vedas or books of knowledge. From Vedic Sanskrit evolved classical Sanskrit which was the basis for Hindu, Buddhist and Jain literature. Sanskrit is thus primarily a language of spiritual knowledge, a revelation of the truth patterns of the cosmic mind. More spiritual teachings and a greater diversity of spiritual concepts and experiences can be found in Sanskrit than in any other language. Hence, it is a good foundation for a global language of consciousness, the language of the spiritual science of the future, as it was the basis for that of the past. It has several important and unique values.

First, it is the oldest form and probable root of the greatest number of languages and the languages spoken by the greatest numbers of people in the world, the Indo-european. These include the main languages of Europe and north India, also many of those of Iran and the Middle East (like Persian, Kurdish or Armenian). Though its grammatical forms are different, it has many common roots with such other important ancient languages as Egyptian or Sumerian. To the east we can find many Sanskrit roots as far away as in the Hawaiian language. Many languages of ancient times, like the Scythian of Central Asia, were also Indo-Iranian in nature.

Second, Sanskrit is the oldest most continually used language in the world and may represent the oldest and most original form of human language. By the most conservative accounts it has been used continuously since 1500 B.C.; by more liberal accounts it was in use before 6000 B.C. Classical Sanskrit follows the same basic patterns since the time of Panini, who probably lived around the time of the Buddha.

Third, it has the largest literature of any language. Along with the sacred literature of two of the world's great religions, Hinduism and

Buddhism, it possesses a larger group of works on spirituality, metaphysics and mythology than any other language. It has an extensive literature of poetry, drama and philosophy, though much has been lost in time.

Fourth, it is the most scientific language. It is the only language devised according to where in the mouth the sounds are made. For this reason most of modern linguistics arose from the reexamination of Sanskrit in the nineteenth century. Grammar, philology and etymology are perhaps more developed in Sanskrit than in any other tongue. It is perhaps the most self-consistent and homogenous of all languages, most others being composites of different languages or dialects.

Sanskrit thus lends itself to be the language of the New Age of global culture. In the future, how many centuries one cannot say, humanity is bound to return to it, at least as its spiritual language or language of learning.

Sanskrit has more words for the Divine and more precise terms for defining consciousness and meditative experience than any other language. It is the language of the higher mind and thereby gives us access to its laws and vibratory structures. It is the language of the Gods, the higher planes of the mind, and affords us access to the powers of these domains.

THE FORM OF THE SANSKRIT LANGUAGE

Sanskrit derives from five primal sounds. These are the vowels *a, i, u* and the semi-vowels *r* and *l*. Each has its characteristic meaning and energetic effect.

a   (pronounced like our word as in the article *a*) is the sound of pure being, existence. It is the infinite, the absolute beyond and behind creation. Its nature is open, expansive, relaxing, affirming.

i   (Pronounced like the *i* in *it*) is the sound of will and consciousness. It is the infinitesimal, the atom, the bindu, the point of pure concentration from which the creation expands. Its action is contracting, directing, desiring, guiding.

u   (Pronounced like the *u* in *put*) is the sound of energy and power. It gives intensity and force, often violence. It is the matrix, the force-field, the vibratory structure behind creation. It gives strength, protection, both gathering things in and warding things away.

r   (A soft or vowel sound *r*, as in *true*) is the sound of order and structure. It gives law, stability and right movement to things. It is the basis of cosmic law and intelligence.

ḷ   (A soft or vowel sound *l̤*) is the sound of form and stability. It gives joy, harmony, contentment, and inertia.

These five basic sounds create the five orders of consonants, which reflect and expand their meaning. The vowel *a* creates the gutturals: *k, kh, g, gh,* and *ṅ (ng)*. The vowel *i* creates the palatals: *c, ch, h, j, jh,* and *ñ (ny* or *gy)*. The vowel *u* creates the labials: *p, ph, b, bh,* and *m.* The sound *r̤* creates the cerebral set (pronounced with the tongue curled back towards the palate) of *ṭ, ṭh, ḍ, ḍh,* and *ṇ.* The sound *ḷ* creates the dental set (pronounced with the tongue behind the teeth) of *t, th, d, dh,* and *n.* These are the twenty-five constants of Sanskrit.

There are sixteen vowels in Sanskrit. The vowels *a, i,* and *u* have short and long forms. The long form of *ā* is pronounced like in *father,* the long form of *ī* as in *sheet,* the long form of *ū* as in *boot.* Combined forms or diphthongs are *e, ai, o,* and *au.* The vowel *e* is pronounced as our long vowel *a* as in *rate.* The vowel *ai* is pronounced as our long vowel *i* as in *site.* The vowel *o* is pronounced as in *home* and *au* as in *ouch.* Long forms of the semi-vowels *r̄* and *ḹ* also exist, though they seldom actually occur. An aspiration of the vowel sound is recognized as the letter *ḥ,* and a nasalization of the vowel sound as the letter *ṁ.*

An intermediate class between the vowels and consonants is the nine semi-vowels and aspirants. These are *y, r, l, v, h, s, ś* (palatal), *ṣ* (cerebral), *kṣ* (the Sanskrit equivalent of the Greek χ).

These fifty letters form the garland of the Goddess, the Kundalini, which is the power of speech. They reside in the different chakras of the subtle body.

In the Upanishads, the series of vowels represents the Spirit or consciousness (Indra). Consonants represent matter or death, as they are based on limitation. A consonant cannot be said without a vowel. The intermediate class of the semi-vowels and aspirants represents the creative power through which Spirit becomes matter (Prajapati).

LANGUAGE AND THE WORD AS A SPIRITUAL PATH

The Vedic Yoga stresses the power of the Word or the Chant. She is defined as the Goddess Vak, Vani or Saraswati. Vak is the word as the power of command. Saraswati is the Goddess of the endless stream of wisdom.

Many different forms of the Yoga of sound exist in Sanskrit literature. According to the Yoga and Sankhya system, sound is the root of all other sensory potentials. It is the sensory quality which belongs to ether, the original element. Hence, through it all the elements can be controlled. The

mind itself is composed of sound. It is the reverberation of our words and
the ideas they represent which forms the pattern of the mind. Hence, a
conscious use of sound both purifies and controls the mind. Most important of the Yogas of sound may be the Shabda Brahma Mantra Yoga of
Bhartrihari (c. 500 A.D.), which describes the understanding of sound as
the highest yoga and the most direct path to the Divine.

These Yogas of sound are not concerned merely with the gross
articulated sounds. Four levels of sound are recognized in Vedic and
Puranic literature. The *Rig Veda (I.164.45.)* states, "Four are the levels of
sound. Three hidden in secrecy cannot be manipulated. Mortals speak
only with the fourth." These four are called Vaikhari, Madhyama,
Pashyanti and Para. Vaikhari dwells in the throat and is our gross,
articulated sound. Madhyama dwells in the heart and is our mental pattern
or idea behind the sound. Pashyanti means seeing. It dwells in the solar
plexus. It is the essential meaning behind the sound, its archetypal content.
Para means the transcendent. It is the essence of all sounds. It dwells in
the root chakra. (Note that the powers of sound dwell in progressively
lower chakras. This is not because they are progressively lower powers
but because they have the power over progressively deeper and more
difficult parts of our nature.)

Hence, the Yoga of sound is meant to take us back from our gross
sounds to their idea content to the perception they represent and ultimately
to the pure being behind that perception. It is not a process of merely
repeating sounds or thinking about words but tracing the origin of sound
and meaning back to awareness itself by the power of meditation.

Sanskrit is the language of mantra, of spiritually empowered sounds.
Its usage is to bring our minds back to the consciousness and power of
mantra. Mantra is not just concerned with sound but with meaning.
According to the view of the Yoga of sound, there is only one meaning in
life, which is the Divine or our own Self. Each thing ultimately means all
things. Each object is a symbol for the universe itself. Words represent
this universal meaning broken down, fragmented and compartmentalized.
To cognize any individual object, we must first recognize its ground of
being, which is the Divine. Yet we fail to notice this as it is immediate and
before the activity of our thought and choice. If we hold to this primacy
of being as the meaning of all objects, all things become doorways to the
infinite.

While ordinary language seeks more precise and differentiated meanings, spiritual languages seek an expanded and integrated comprehension
until one is all and all is one. They aim to free meaning from its
imprisonment in words and their arbitrary conventions. In reality, all
things are meaningless in themselves, or each thing means the entire

universe. It is only the universality of meaning which allows for specific meanings to occur. This inquiry into meaning is the essence of the Yoga of sound. It involves freeing our mind from its attachment to particular sounds and to the tyranny of names.

The Tantric system also has an important Sound Yoga. It is best developed in the Kashmiri Shaiva works of Abhinavagupta (c. 1100 A.D.). Sound is the body of the Goddess who is the Yoga Shakti or power of Yoga. Sound thus creates the current of force which lifts us into the infinite.

THE IMPORTANCE OF MANTRA

Mantra has become well known in the West. We normally associate it, rather superficially, with some meaningless sound we repeat mechanically until we are put in some kind of trance. Actually, mantra is quite different than this.

All learning involves the energization of the mind. It is by the power of attention, the concentration of the mind, that we come to know anything. As long as we are distracted or our minds are wandering, we cannot come to really see anything. Hence, the real object of learning is not to learn anything in particular but to gain the mastery of the mind through the power of attention. Then we can find truth in all things.

This energization of the mind is the true purpose and meaning of mantra. Whenever we have a deep insight or profound realization in life, that thought has a special power. The empowered thought is mantra. Hence, the more deeply we can think and inquire into things, the more our thoughts become mantra; the greater our power of observation, the more mantric force enters into our minds.

Just as the practice of Yoga requires a special power or Yoga Shakti to facilitate it, so does the practice of mantra require a special Mantra Shakti for it to be effective. This is a conscious and creative energization of sound and meaning. It is something like the difference between poetry and ordinary speech. For mantra to work it must have at least as much creative empowerment as a good poem. To bring about this empowerment requires a special concentration of the mind. It may be aided by the grace of a teacher, by the power of an initiation. It may come from within by the power of our own insight, aspiration and connection with the inner guide. But without this creative vision behind the mantra, mantra may be no more than a form of self-hypnosis.

When this energization of speech occurs, we begin to find profound meanings in a few simple sounds. Sound becomes meaning, and we do not need an idea to interpret the sounds of the mind. Such primary sounds as Om give rise to whole fields or spectrums of meaning. They break down

the barrier of language and take us into the universal state of communication which is silence and peace.

The main mantras of Hinduism and Buddhism all derive from Sanskrit. While mantras need not be in Sanskrit, it lends itself more easily to
the mantric approach than other languages because it originates from
mantra. Other languages require overcoming their inertia, their less conscious structure, to facilitate the energy of the mantra.

Mantras are of two types: longer chants and shorter seed-syllables.
Most known are the shorter seed or bija-mantras like Om. These consist
of various root sounds like Om, Hum or Shrim. It is from these root sounds
that the entire Sanskrit language is evolved and into which it can be
reduced. These roots develop into both nouns and verbs. For example,
from the root 'ta', meaning to extend, there develops nouns like 'tala', the
palm of the hand, or verbs like 'tanoti', he extends.

Longer mantras are chants, like the Vedic verses, of which the Gayatri
is most important. They are more like prayers and show language in its
developed form.

The shorter root mantras have a more universal meaning. We can use
them according to their energetics even if we do not understand the
language that develops from them.

The longer chants depend more upon our sense of their meaning and
our intentions. They can be more easily translated into ordinary language
as such prayers for universal peace, as "may all beings be happy."

PRIMARY MANTRAS
Om

Om is said to be the essence of all mantras, the highest of all mantras,
the Divine Word or Shabda Brahman itself. Om is said to be the essence
of the Vedas. One need not know or study the Vedas, one need only chant
Om. Om is the sound of the infinite. It gives power to all mantras. Hence,
all mantras begin and end with Om and without it are said to be deprived
of power. Om itself clears the mind for meditation.

Om consists of three sounds; the vowel *a*, the vowel *u* and the
nasalized *m* sound. Hence, it is sometimes written as Aum (or as Alm at
the beginning of the *Koran,* as Arabic *l* is often pronounced as *u* when it
comes before another consonant).

The three portions of Aum relate to the states of waking, dream and
deep sleep and to the three gunas of rajas, sattva and tamas. They are ruled
by the Gods Brahma, Vishnu and Shiva, the Divine in its threefold role
as the creator, sustainer and destroyer of the universe.

In the Vedas, Om is the sound of the Sun, the sound of light. It is the sound of assent (affirmation) and ascent (it has an upwards movement and uplifts the soul, as the sound of the Divine eagle or falcon).

Hum

Hum (pronounced as in our word *whom*) is the sound of Divine wrath. It destroys all negativity. It is a Shiva sound and a sound of Agni, the Divine Fire, through which all the other Gods or Divine powers can be invoked. As Om is the sound of the individual merging into the infinite, Hum is the sound of the infinite manifesting itself in the individual. It is important in Tibetan Buddhism and among the Sufis as Hu.

Ram

Ram (with a long *a* sound as in *father*) is the sound of Divine light, grace and protection. It gives strength, peace and compassion. It relates to the avatar Rama.

Shrim

Shrim (pronounced *shreem*) is the mantra of beauty, grace, prosperity and abundance and relates to the Goddess. It brings about the fulfillment of all wishes, higher or lower.

Aim

Aim (pronounced *aym*) is the sound of wisdom and relates to Saraswati, the Goddess of knowledge. It increases our powers of attention, concentration, reason and contemplation. It is also the sound of the guru, the spiritual teacher, and brings into play the learning power of the higher mind.

Ma

Ma is the first of all sounds, the name of the Mother. Through this sound we connect with the power and grace of the Divine Mother and her love, nourishment and contentment giving energy.

So'ham

Soham is the natural sound of the breath. So is inhalation and Ham is exhalation. If we breathe deeply and listen to the sound of our breath we hear these sounds. In Sanskrit the root 'sa' from which 'so' develops means to hold, to have power, to be. It gives inspiration and power. 'Ham' means to leave, abandon, cast out, hence to expel or exhale.

If we eliminate the consonants from Soham, we get Om. So is Shakti and Ham is Shiva. Through them we balance the God and the Goddess within ourselves. So'ham pranayama is natural deep breathing with attention to the sound of these mantras.

The Gayatri Mantra

From the mantra Om develops the Gayatri mantra, a longer mantra or chant. Its translation is:

> "Om, We meditate upon the adorable effulgence of the Divine
> Creative Sun that he may give impulse to our intelligence."

The Divine Creative Sun is Savitar, the Divine Father and guide of the yogic movement of life. He is a form of Vishnu. This mantra is chanted by the twice-born, those reborn in the truth of the unity of consciousness, at the rising and setting of the Sun. It is for celebrating the miracle of Divine light outwardly and inwardly and aligning our intelligence with the evolutionary power inherent in nature.

THE USE OF MANTRA

Mantras are perhaps the most important tools for clearing and cleansing the mind. Mantra helps break up our unconscious and subconscious thought and desire patterns which keep us in bondage to past conditioning. If we observe ourselves we see that all day long there is a background chatter in the mind. It may be the repetition of some song we have heard on the radio, it may be a rehashing of some experience we have just had, an insult or argument for example, or a consideration of what we are about to do, but all the time this background noise is going on. It forms the field of our thoughts and serves to drain away our energy of attention.

It is usually not possible for us to directly silence the mind. Our mind is too divided and we have too many unresolved conflicts. It is, however, always within our power to chant a mantra. If we do this regularly, above all, if it becomes our primary mental activity, it gradually replaces this background noise of the mind. Instead of hearing an old song or childhood experience reverberating behind our surface mind, we hear the mantra; Om, Ram, Hare Krishna or whatever it may be. Our subconscious is restructured by the energy of the mantra and ceases to resist the intentions of our conscious mind to meditate. This is the right use of the mantra.

Rightly employed mantras can be used to clear negative emotions from the mind. The mantra Hum, for example, eliminates fear. The mantra Ram gives peace.

Hence, mantra is also an important part of Yoga psychology. It is the main Yogic tool for deconditioning the mind. It does not require any elaborate psychoanalysis but only an ongoing practice. Through it we can change the structure of the mind that allows psychological problems to exist in the first place. In this way we change the nature of the mind rather than merely analyze it (which does not have the power to fundamentally change it anyway). As long as our thoughts are not mantric we are bound to have some emotional problems in life. The solution is not to study our emotions but to practice the mantra. It is the personal or egoistic energization of the mind which causes mental suffering. The spiritual energization of the mind through mantra is the antidote.

Mantra thus leads us to meditation and silence. It is not an end in itself to repeat a sound. Hence, we should remain open after our repetition of the mantra to that stillness of mind and learn to dwell in it. That is where the Om vibration leads us. The sound of the waves merges us back into the silent depths of the ocean.

VEDIC AND CLASSICAL SANSKRIT

It is mainly classical Sanskrit that is studied and in which most Sanskrit texts are written. But it is in the older Vedic language that the real power of Sanskrit lies hidden. The Vedic language gives the Divine Word and is intuitive in nature. The classical language is often highly intellectual and, though much more profound than other languages, seldom has the richness and creativity of the Vedic. Hence, for really learning Sanskrit or the language of mantra, it is important to study the Vedic language. In it is perhaps the key to all language and to the thought process of the Divine Mind.

The most basic form of Sanskrit is the seed-syllables or bija mantras like Om. We can observe these in their original form behind the words of the Vedas. In the Vedic language they are still alive and interrelated. In the later language they retire into the background as custom gains a greater role in the meaning of words. In Tantric texts they are given separately, and their action on the different parts of our nature is precisely described. These seed-syllables are not so much a part of a spoken language as a way of energizing the mind. As such, they are universal and not limited to any particular spoken dialect, though all languages ultimately derive from them. We can learn them without learning the Sanskrit language or its grammar. In this way we can access the power of mantra without getting caught in the complexity of language.

7
KARMA AND THE SCIENCE
OF REBIRTH

KARMA

Karma is one of the most commonly known but poorly understood concepts of Vedic Science. The term first occurs in the Vedas themselves which refer to karma as the ritual we do in life. In the Vedic view all life is a ritual; that is, all life is a repeated action which produces certain subtle or occult results. It is these results which determine our future condition and the state of the world we live in. Each action has a certain effect which determines who we are and what we will become. Our most constant and intended action, our daily practice, thereby is the measure of the direction of the evolution of our soul and our effect upon the world-soul. Whatever this may be, whether it is making money or seeking truth, this is our worship or way of directing our energies in life and must have certain consequences. In the Upanishads this secret doctrine of karma and rebirth is first explained in rational and philosophical terms.

Any sensitive person is struck by the amount of injustice there is in the world. Most of the time, we see those who are evil triumph over those who are good. We often see the good man suffer in poverty or social rejection, while the man of evil or mixed character is rewarded with money, fame and power. Saints, sages and avatars are often ignored, slandered or martyred. We observe that the positions people hold in life seldom correspond to their inner qualities. Men of real leadership qualities are seldom found in positions of leadership. Men of true wisdom are seldom found at the head of educational institutes. Most religious leaders lack in any real spiritual experience.

While we do see instances wherein evil men fall or are defeated by the good, it appears more as an exception than the rule. We see a world teeming with inequality, wherein the weak and poor are often trampled under. Today, the earth itself is being destroyed, along with much of its plant and animal populations. It appears that if there is a God, he is not watching over this world and is not involved with its evolution.

The doctrine of karma, by the common understanding, means "as you sow, so shall you reap." By this many take it to mean that those who are rich and affluent in life must be reaping the rewards of past good actions, while those who are poor and destitute are paying back for previous misdeeds.

Such attitudes of karma are simplistic and erroneous because karma is based upon the inner reality of things, not upon the outer names and forms of the world. Karma, as a spiritual law, is not adjusted according to our various and conflicting cultural definitions of success and failure. Our life and consciousness is like an iceberg, the greater portion of it lies beneath the waters of our ordinary awareness. As long as we only judge the visible portion of things we will come to many wrong conclusions about reality. Karma, as a spiritual law, must apply to the whole reality of man, not just to the preconceptions or prejudices of the surface mind and emotions.

From such an inner standpoint, the soul's happiness is often the suffering of the ego, and the happiness of the ego is often the suffering of the soul. In this regard good fortune in life may be a sign of a strong ego, while suffering may occur to us to awaken us to the truth behind the outer forms of things. More evolved souls may choose more difficult incarnations, while less evolved souls may require comfort and ease. It is like mountain climbers. The beginners must take only the easy slope, while the experienced go after difficult inclines.

We also see that anyone who chooses the spiritual life is going against the outer order of society. Hence, it is usual for a spiritual aspirant to receive criticism or undergo hardship from the outer world. According to the ancient myths, all the Gods abandon us so that we can discover ourselves; only we ourselves can destroy the dragon of our own ignorance. Oppression or hardship in life may not be an indication of bad karma but the shadow of the good grace of the spiritual path in a world that is contrary to it. Moreover, the spiritual life often involves a quickening of our karma, an attempt to work it out at a faster rate. For this reason we may experience more negative karma as we move along the path. This, again, is no indication of necessary evil in our nature but part of a process of purification.

Ultimately, we must go beyond all karma, good or evil. This is to place our sense of reality in our true Self, not in the effects of our actions. We must eventually renounce the fruit of all our actions. In that alone is freedom and transcendence. Hence, the highest good is motiveless and does not seek results. The greatest virtue does not seek to change the world or improve ourselves but to rest in harmony with the peace of what is.

CAUSE AND EFFECT

Karma is a natural law, not a moral law. If we put our hands into a fire and get burned, it is because we have violated natural law. We have acted contrary to the inherent qualities of things. There is no God who forbids us to touch fire and who burns us to punish us for violating his dictate. Just as there is natural law in the outer world, so does natural law apply to the realm of emotion and thought. Unfortunately, we are not as perceptive in the inner or psychological realm as in the outer. We do not always see how we are hurting ourselves through the violation of our own emotional nature. All bad or evil thoughts and emotions must first hurt ourselves, as our mind is their field of manifestation. If I am angry, that anger must first affect me, not only disturbing my emotions and thoughts, but harming my physical body as well. I may blame another for it, but I am still creating it in myself and have to experience the consequences of it within my own psyche.

The relationship between cause and effect may not appear as dramatically or immediately in the inner world, as it does in the outer. When I put my hand in a fire, I feel quite directly the mistake I have committed. When I give my mind over to a fiery emotion like anger or hatred, I may not make the same ascertainment. Moreover, should I take advantage of another person, for example, abuse their friendship, I might not know what this means until someone does the same thing to me. We are simply not aware of cause and effect in the mind, partly because we are not trained to do so. In fact we are encouraged to ignore it. If we can make an unfair amount of money on someone, as long as it is legal, we feel we have gotten away with it. Though we may have gotten away with it in the outer world, in the inner world we cannot escape the consequence of that action. The prime result of all wrong actions, all actions which cause harm to others or increase falsehood and illusion in the world, is that they bar us from entering the inner realms of the mind. They shut the door on the inner realm of being, consciousness and bliss in which is our only true and lasting fulfillment. Though we may gain in the outer world, even if we gain it all, we still lose the inner realm, compared to which the outer is a mere shadow or bubble.

Hence, it is important for us to note the cause and effect relationship between our actions in time. We can easily adjust to what has an immediate effect, but we do not always see how we are experiencing the results of what we have done in the more distant past. If we eat bad food, we may develop an ulcer in time. But we are more aware of the immediate taste of the food, which may be pleasing to the senses, and so do not connect our disease with its cause, which only manifests later. As long as we fail to trace the causes of our actions back to their origin, as long as we are unable to see the chain of time, we will create our own suffering. Some of these causes may come from previous lives and be lost in the dark night of time, but we can be sure they are there.

The law of karma does not mean simply that we will be rewarded or punished in the future for the effect of actions done today. Its main effect is immediate. The law of karma states that the condition of our consciousness and inner happiness is based upon how we act in the present. The main punishment for an evil man is that he has to reside in the consciousness of evil, which cuts himself off from his true soul and source of life. The reward of true virtue is that it puts us in contact with the eternal and with a sense of well-being transcending outer circumstances. In this regard, evil is its own punishment and virtue its own reward. By this immediate effect any action causes us to abide in the state of consciousness which produced it. Evil actions cause us to remain in a state of evil or petty mindedness. Good actions give us added energy to remain in a state of peace.

Yet true good, we must remember, is always unpremeditated. We should follow the good for its own sake, not to get the reward of good karma. Those who seek rewards remain trapped in the surface of life and give emphasis to outer over inner values. Action done with the intent to gain is already evil, though it may be seeking the goal of enlightenment.

In this regard we must remember that most of the evil in the world is done in the name of goodness. It is in the name of religion or political idealism that the most violence has been done in this world. We all want to do what is good. It is the nature of the soul to seek the good. No one will consciously do something they think is bad. The problem is our concept of good is limited or selfish, or we feel that we can impose it on others. What is good for us may not be good for everyone else. Any action that is imposing our idea of what is good or true upon others is in fact evil, because it is a violation of the freedom and integrity of the soul. Fanaticism and self-righteousness are the most evil of things. For this reason the Vedic teaching does not try to spread itself through seeking converts, nor does it encourage any form of propaganda.

Most of our own sins or mistakes in life are done out of an effort to be good or to please others. Whenever we attempt to conform to an external standard of what is good, we may lose contact with the real internal source of good, which is our true Self and soul, our inner connection with the Divine. The outer good is a social convention, not the true good of our soul. Only when we are willing to follow what is truly good inside ourselves will we have a beneficent presence or action in life. As long as we act to please others, we will remain slaves of the external world and under the power of external influences, which is the real evil. Hence, to pursue what is of true good we may have to risk the disfavor of family, friends and the social order. This does not mean we must rebel against these influences and seek to go against them. It means our action must be based upon the universal and the eternal, which is not limited to an external standard.

The real law is that whatever is not good for our soul cannot be good for the souls of others either. To cater to the ego needs of others is not good for us and harms them as well.

True good, therefore, cannot be measured by how much people like us, how much money we have given to charity, or by how good the world thinks we are. According to the Vedas, the highest good is to be ourselves, to rest in our true Self or inner nature apart from all external influences and motivations. This allows for the flow of Divine grace into the world wherein we go beyond all the superficial appearances of good and evil. Great beings bless the world by their mere existence and need not do any other action to uplift humanity.

What is necessary, therefore, is not that we do good karma but that we are true to ourselves, to our deepest Self. Both good and bad karma bind the soul, just as a golden chain can bind a man as much as an iron one. It is usually easier to go from good karma to beyond karma, but some instances of great yogis have occurred wherein their early part of life involved bad karma, even the working of black magic or criminal deeds. No one should be judged. Any soul can turn around and move to the truth. In fact, it is often the self-righteous who have the most difficult time for in self-righteousness we lose the capacity to see our faults and limitations and thereby are unable to grow.

In the Vedic system, there is no ultimate evil, only ignorance. Even the most evil person operates out of a false or perverted sense of the good. We should not hate them. They are merely a manifestation of the negative thoughts we collectively project. What we need to do is to create an atmosphere of understanding in life wherein the soul in children is not perverted by fear and desire. Then, most negative karma will not have a field in which it can grow.

The law of karma means that the other is also our self. Whatever we do to others, we do to ourselves. Our karmas are all linked together with collective as well as individual karma. Yet, even if we transcend our individual karma, we cannot change the collective karma or the nature of the world. Each soul has to grow for itself and must be free to gain the experiences it needs.

Karma teaches us that there is an absolute inner justice in life which cannot be violated, even by the grossest injustice of the outer world. Suffering and misfortune teach us to look deeper and see the real state of things. Without them we would probably not grow inwardly but would relax into lives of superficiality and dissipation. We should welcome difficulties as our friends and teachers. Suffering is the way of spiritual growth for human beings. It should not be taken as a simple indication of bad karma but as a means to take us beyond karma.

As long as we are content with what we can achieve in the realm of action, we cannot find what is real in life. Being itself, which is truth, cannot be arrived at through action. It is not a result that any action can produce. The highest action is to give up attachment to our actions and to act only insofar as we are prompted by our inner being. Thus, we must not take good karma to be an end in itself or be content with it. Good and bad karma are the light and shadow in the mirror but our true nature is the mirror, and to know it we must not be overcome by good or bad reflections within it.

REBIRTH

Rebirth is also a well known, but seldom really understood, term from the Vedas. It is often called reincarnation, but this can be misleading. The ego we know and experience is not reborn. The personality of this particular incarnation is not particularly stable even within it. Most of us change significantly the idea of who we are several times in life. We cannot expect it to go on to another. Nor is our inner Self ever born, nor does it die, as its nature is eternal. The true reincarnating entity is the causal body, wherein our karmic impressions are stored. It is its stream of impressions that continues with the reflection of consciousness upon it, but there never is any real separate self. The individual is only a power of Divine aspiration and service.

Many ask, if reincarnation is a fact, how can the population continue to increase? Today there are many more times as many people as there were at any other stage in history. Where have all the souls suddenly come from?

Neither the inner Self nor the causal body is a quantifiable entity. There is not a simple correspondence of one soul or causal body per physical body. The inner world does not follow the same logic as the outer world. A great enlightened individual may hold within himself a greater spiritual force than millions of people. It is also possible for one soul to take more than one birth at the same time, either high or low. A greater population does, however, tend to decrease the quality of the soul or the soul power in incarnation and spreads it more thin.

The process of death is like an extended version of the process of sleep. At death we enter into a deeper sleep. This takes us first into a state of greater dream. We enter more directly and completely into the astral plane, which we touch in the dream state. There, we experience various positive or negative mental states according to our knowledge and action in life. Our predominant mental conditions arise as the impressions we have gathered in life are released. We may see the friends and relatives we have most thought about in life. We may go to various positive or negative astral worlds, the basis of the ideas of heaven and hell. These usually reflect our religious conditioning, as they are the reflections of our thoughts. A Christian will experience a Christian heaven or hell, a Muslim a Muslim heaven or hell. These are all temporary. Sometimes the heavens are based more on illusion and wrong thinking than the hells. We gradually move through the astral plane until we come to the causal plane. Our consciousness enters into the soul and therein rests and gathers the materials for a new incarnation.

Less evolved souls may only experience a prolonged deep sleep between incarnations. Very advanced souls may enter into a deep meditative trance (the level of the causal world) and may reincarnate quickly. Souls of intermediate development may spend much time on the different levels of the astral planes to assimilate their life experience. Causal experience is of a deep formless meditative nature. Through it we extract the essence of our experience and understand the laws of life from a position transcending time.

Less evolved souls usually incarnate into the same location on earth and seek a similar life-experience. More evolved souls may take on quite different life-experiences or incarnate in different lands. There is no specific rule; as usual, it depends upon the need of the individual. It is not the ego that chooses its incarnation. It is the soul. It determines these not by an action of will or thought as is known to us, but by the natural impulse of its energies and aspirations. The soul does not cognize name and form. It does not say, "let me be born in a poor family in China and work my way up as a doctor." It moves according to the current of energy it projects, and from that, the particular circumstances of the birth arise.

Many of the versions of rebirth and after death states we find presented in various books and teachings are products of the imagination of people. The soul is presented like a person reviewing his past actions and planning his future according to some master plan. Such stories only serve to encourage the manipulations of the mind, not to bring us into the state of peace and natural spontaneous harmony. The true soul is beyond the mind and does not function through thought. It envisions things but as an unfoldment of the heart, not a structure of thought.

LIBERATION

The goal of the soul in evolution is mergence into the Divine or the inner Self. This brings about freedom from the cycle of rebirth (samsara). This is the highest goal of human life through which everything is accomplished. It can be brought about only through Self-knowledge. All life is an experience to provide us with Self-knowledge. To see our Self in all beings and all beings in our Self is the essence of life. Only by becoming all can we go beyond all.

Some say that the great Yogis merge into the Unborn and leave the world, leaving others behind without compassion to gain their own personal liberation. This idea shows a great lack of understanding. Liberation is only possible by merging into the Self of all, by becoming one with everything. There is no separate self left over who could leave the world behind or who could act to help it out. Merging into the Self also means merging into the Divine. God is always there to help the souls in the world. So too, the souls merged in him are always there as needed.

Liberation from the world, therefore, is not abandoning the world but merging into the world and beyond, becoming the all. It is a return to our true nature. Hence, from the highest standpoint there is no birth and no death, no one who is born and no one who dies, there is only the unborn, perfect and infinite Self-nature, beyond all limitations and possessed of all powers of self-manifestation.

This state has been called Nirvana, Kaivalya, Mukti, Moksha, etc. It is beyond all states of body and mind and not limited by them. It is everything and nothing, everyone and no one.

KARMA IN VEDIC SCIENCE

All branches of Vedic Science teach us to take control of our karma. This occurs by becoming aware of it. Once we see how we create our destiny, we will avoid the factors which bring us pain. Ayurveda teaches us to discern how, in our physical existence, our actions done out of harmony with our constitution must breed disease. Vedic astrology shows us how we can discern the planetary energies behind our karma and use them as means of liberation from it. Rituals aid us in warding off the effects of collective and individual karmic imbalances. Yet Yoga and meditation is the sovereign means of going beyond karma. It teaches us through detachment how to no longer be affected by karma. This is the means of bringing our karmic bondage to an end. Then, as the Upanishads say, "we are free to act as we will in all the worlds."

Freedom from karma is not incapacity but the highest accomplishment and greatest mastery over all the domains of life. The key to it is not to seek. Our inner Self is the central point of the universe. We need not act overtly. If we merely abide in our own deepest nature, all the universe must respond to it, must revolve around it. All things are accomplished by their own nature, and in that nature is peace in both action and non-action. Karma is based upon desire. It reflects the freedom of our soul. As long as we have desires, we must take embodiment to fulfill them. As desire is limited, has a specific aim, it must have an end or lead to sorrow. Hence, only when we desire everything or nothing will we find peace. Yoga aims at going beyond desire. This does not mean giving up the things we want but seeing that it is beneath our dignity as a Divine being to want anything or make our happiness dependent upon anything that comes from the outside.

8
UNIVERSAL FORMS OF WORSHIP
TEMPLES, PUJA AND HOMA

According to the ancient seers and yogis, Nature herself is the manifest form of the deity. All things in nature in their true reality are objects of worship, forms of the sacred. We live in the sacred, mysterious and magical. It is only the mind that makes things profane or devoid of spiritual meaning; our sense of familiarity which misses the uniqueness of each thing and each moment. Each thing is in its true nature a name and form of the Divine. It is only our utilitarian vision that makes them otherwise. For this reason the best form of worship is to take a walk or a retreat in nature. Many sacred places exist in nature, and one is always accessible to us. Mother Nature is the Divine Mother and in her presence is always the upliftment of the soul.

Originally, in human culture, the deities represented the great cosmic powers of nature: the sun, wind, fire and waters. These were seen, not just as material forces, but as Divine powers at work in the world. They also exist inside us as the forces of our body and mind, our breath and perception. Life itself is a form of worship; that is, it is a movement in transcendence, a seeking of ever greater growth and aspiration. The trees are a symbol of the opening up of the life-force to the heaven of truth. The flowers show the unfoldment of love, with its beauty, color and fragrance. The sky shows the expanse of the cosmic mind. The ocean shows the depth of Divine feeling. All nature is the language of God and proclaims the Divine word. It is only when we link up to the fact of the worship which is life itself that we are truly in a state of prayer, and that we are really alive at all.

TEMPLES
We also need more formal places of worship as we no longer live in nature. The Divine presence should not be excluded from our communities. Temples are important, as they provide a sacred space for the community to gather wherein our spiritual energies can be renewed. They serve as channels to bring Divine grace into the world. They become a focus for our collective aspiration. Each temple should be the meeting

place for the whole community wherein we come together to share our aspiration in life.

Temples, moreover, are not connected only with the physical nature. They are linked to nature on the astral plane. Hence, they use forms of art, color, sound and incense which bring us into the presence and power of the subtle nature. They become doorways into the subtle realms of religion and spirituality.

Temples serve to create an occult force in the world. They keep our psyche and collective mind clear and open to Divine grace. They serve as a focus to bring the energy of the sacred into our sphere of activity. As such, they aid in the prevention of social calamities like crime, wars or plagues. As we have few real temples to protect us anymore, this leaves our societies vulnerable on a subtle level to the negative forces of the subconscious and the negative effects of our wrong actions. We can judge the nature of any society by the nature of its temples or churches. However, it is not their mere number but the quality of aspiration projected through them which reveals this. It is not enough to make rich and opulent temples, though to the Divine we should offer what is most valuable to us. What is more important is that we see the Divine everywhere, that the temple is a presence we take into our whole sphere of action in society and we treat each being as sacred.

Each house should be a temple, as worship is the natural center for human life. Hence, in each house we should have some central altar, some place of meditation or prayer, enhanced perhaps by some form of the Divine or sacred object from nature, if but a flower. So too, each family should have a central form of worship like a daily chant, prayer or meditation. This need not be formal or rigid. It is the expression of the heart which is the most important thing. Without this we have no true family, no common soul, but are only a collection of separate personalities with no sacrament to link us together. There is so much truth and beauty in each one of us that it is sad we spend our times trapped in external forms of entertainment, when we should be sharing our souls with each other. Any human being we live with is a divinity to be cherished. And within ourselves, above all, is the place where that Divinity is to be enshrined. For this we also need time alone so that our individual connection with the Divine is pure and direct.

A temple, however, is different than our more usual idea of a church. In a temple teachings may be given but there should be no preaching. We should encourage each individual to awaken to the Divine in their own way, not seek to impose a particular pattern upon them. A temple is a space of openness which allows for the individual to find God or truth within themselves. It is open to all truth, expressed perhaps through a specific form, but it is not a monument to a particular belief as against others. If that space of openness is violated, the power of the temple goes with it.

Temples should be made to all possible manifestations of the Divine according to the Divine potential in each form and each aspect of nature. In India the Divine is worshipped in animal forms, but not because animals are worshipped. It is to aid us in seeing the Divine presence in the animal kingdom. Temples may also include reverence to great teachers of the past. This is to link us with our common humanity and the great stream of human aspiration through history, not to attach us to personalities of the past. Hence, the basis of the true temple is freedom. A temple should be made to freedom of worship, not dedicated to preserving only one form of belief. The true temples of India have this free spirit about them.

The body itself is the main temple of the deity which is consciousness itself. If we do not maintain this inner temple, it is of little value to honor the outer. In the practise of Yoga this inner temple is the seat of worship which is the practise of meditation. The temple is the body of the deity made manifest. So too, the body is the temple of the deity made manifest.

DEVOTIONAL WORSHIP
PUJA

The main form of worship used in the Vedic and Yogic teaching is temple worship, attending the pujas or ritual worship of the Gods and Goddesses. Pujas are short rituals and consist of chants, flowers, lamps, incense and food and water, etc. offered to the Divine, usually in the form of a statue enshrined in the temple. Puja itself means flower offering. It symbolizes the natural opening of the heart to the Divine the way a flower naturally unfolds its petals. Pujas are to be done with the same purity, openness, receptivity and innocence, a spontaneous updwelling of our innate love of life.

The seers saw in this flower offering the natural form of worship, nature's ultimate expression of love of God, and they sought to embody it in our human lives. Flowers are relatively new comers to evolution and parallel the evolution of mammals. They are the vegetable kingdom's counterpart of devotion. Hence, they link us up to the aspiration of Nature herself, to the Divine's seeking of the Divine in its own creative play.

Pujas are done regularly several times a day. They are far more informal than any church service, and watching them takes but a few minutes. Pujas can also be done in one's home. Many are simple enough to do oneself. More complicated pujas may require a trained priest, but in the Vedic Dharma what we do for ourselves is usually considered better than what we have others do for us, as it is the Self itself which is the Divine. Often a puja is no more than lighting a ghee lamp before a deity. It is usually one's own personal worship, however imperfect, that is best, as it alone can provide an opening to the Divine within.

Usually puja is combined with meditation, as meditation is the primary mode of inner worship. Puja purifies our environment, our senses and emotions to allow for a deeper meditation in the mind. Hence, after any puja we should sit and meditate if but for a moment.

THE FIRE OFFERING
HOMA

Another important practise is homa, the fire offering. Homa is more ancient than puja. It comes from Vedic times when fire was the main resource used in life. Each house was built around a central fire. Each community had its central or communal fire. Such fires were continued unextinguished for generations. Some first enkindled thousands of years ago are still burning today. Not only do we find this worship of fire in the Vedic teachings, the Persians worshipped fire and the modern Zoroastrians in both India and Iran still have their ancient fires burning. Ancient Rome had a similar cult of fire carried on by the vestal virgins, as did most of the ancient European peoples. These fires served to link the different communities and families in a common aspiration. They provided a link with the souls of those who came before and those who are to come.

Fire is the Divine presence, the presence of light in the material world. No better symbol for the Divine can be found. The spirit is hidden in all material things the way fire is latent in wood. Hence, fire is our most convenient symbol of the Divine and our aspiration towards it. In the homa ceremony we offer our thoughts and emotions to the Divine. We sacrifice the impurities of our lower nature into the Fire of awareness. We can write down our failings in life or the things in our nature we wish to be corrected and offer them into such a sacred fire. This will align us with the powers of nature and the spirit to correct them. Or we can offer into the fire those higher goals and blessings we wish to bring about. It will also serve to energize them. Fire is the Divine messenger. Whatever we offer to it is taken to the Divine and comes back with the portion of Divine energy we open ourselves to.

What makes a fire sacred is not so much a ritual but the consciousness with which we empower it, the awareness of the sacred we project in and through it.

Whereas puja worships the Divine with form, homa worships the Divine without form. Fire is the symbol of the formless Divine. Whereas puja aims at the opening of the heart, homa aims at awakening the mind and consciousness. Puja is a more feminine form of worship, while homa is more masculine.

In these pujas and homas various offerings are given not only to the Divine but to all forms of life for universal peace and well-being. The most basic prayer is for universal peace and happiness. May all beings be happy, may all beings find peace, is the best prayer. This giving of wishes or blessings is an integral part, the beginning and end of all rituals. It comes with Om, which means all is the Divine, the Self is the Divine. Such worship is not a custom or a religious bias but an expression of the universal truth, an actualization of the universal law, a harmonization with the movement of all life towards the Divine. Such rituals should be done by all according to their nature. They are the essence of true human culture and need not be denied because they do not appear modern or entertaining. Their action is the creative play of the cosmic being which is the true being of man. It is only when we become cosmic and live in harmony with the universe that we are truly human.

Today, we still need these forms of worship in our society. We may adapt them, but their action is an essential part of all human life. Without worship we fail as human beings. Without a collective form of worship we fail as a human society. Through the manifold forms of Hinduism we can bring a universality to our patterns of worship. Without that our religions will only serve to divide us. Worship is an extension of our nature. It is the essence of human nature. It is as spontaneous as our love of nature. The division between nature and the Divine is not a product of truth but of a limited and warped medieval mentality. Once this division between nature and the church is removed, we will find aspiration as easy as play. This does not mean to reduce the spiritual to the crude forms of nature. It means to attune ourselves with the spiritual aspiration inherent in nature and in our own deepest nature.

THE USE OF IMAGES

In oriental religions many images, statues and idols, are used in worship. This has caused the charge of idolatry to be levelled against them by western religions. Islam, Judaism and Protestant Christianity reject all usage of images and consider those who use them to be religiously primitive.

Yet in Hinduism the use of images is only one of many forms of worship. More strongly than western religions, it also emphasizes the formless or impersonal Divine. Besides the gross form or image of the deity, subtle geometric and sound and light forms are used as well. The gross image is just one aspect in directing the mind inward, as well as an aid to seeing the Divine in the forms of life. Many people in the dharmic traditions use no images of any kind. It is not that Hinduism is characterized by idolatry so much as it allows the imagistic and naturalistic approach to the Divine along with all the others.

Images are forms of art, paintings, and sculpture. They serve to draw the artistic mind to the Divine and connect up our creative and spiritual natures. They aid in the concentration of our mental and emotional energies to the Divine. Religions that deny the use of this creative access to the Divine are incomplete. They separate God from nature, man from God and man from man. They do not allow for the spiritualization of the world or the human realization of the Divine. A culture which does not use all forms of art to glorify or access the Divine is not yet mature.

There is thus a scientific way to use images to draw out the deeper powers and potentials of our psyche. We learn to see in the human appearance the indwelling divinity. We learn to see that we are all no more than images or appearances of a deeper Divine consciousness. In this way most of us can benefit spiritually through the right use of images, though it is certainly not the only way to develop our inner potentials.

9

VEDIC COSMOLOGY

THE MULTIDIMENSIONAL UNIVERSE

A conspicuous branch of non-being mortals regard as
the Supreme.   *– Atharva Veda X. 7. 21.*

Modern science has expanded our horizons on the universe. In western culture up to recent times we used to think that the universe was largely confined to this earth and that it had been in existence for less than six thousand years. However, the Vedic and Puranic teaching has always dated our universe as existing for many billions of years, much more so than modern science yet acknowledges. It sees the present universe as just one in a series of manifestations, each marked by an equal period of dissolution (pralaya) wherein no manifestation occurs.

According to the cosmology of yoga, our present view of the universe is still very limited. We are only aware of one plane of existence and though we have and continue to explore it in great detail, in the process we are ignoring or missing the greater part of reality, particularly that which resides within our own deeper consciousness. There are other levels of existence, other dimensions wherein different types of worlds exist much different than our physical realm.

According to the many ancient teachings, including the Vedas, the universe consists of seven levels or planes, of which we are mainly aware of only the first and lowest. These are different densities of reality from gross matter to pure Spirit. They are described as follows:

The Seven Planes of the Universe

1. Food, Sanskrit Anna; the material world and the physical body.

2. Breath or Life, Prana; the vital world and the vital sheath.

3. Emotion, Manas; the emotional world or emotional sheath.

4. Intelligence, Vijnana; the world of intelligence or the intelligence sheath.

5. Bliss, Ananda; the world of bliss or the bliss sheath.

6. Consciousness, Cit.

7. Being, Sat.

Being and Consciousness have no sheath or no world because they transcend manifestation, being immaterial. Hence, though there are seven planes there are only five sheaths.

These seven planes are states of consciousness. It is the same consciousness operating on all of them. It gradually unfolds its powers from the lowest to the highest. These are the seven densities consciousness assumes in its manifestation. They exist not only within us as deeper aspects of our being but each has its own native plane and worlds which are composed of its type of matter (again with the exception of the highest two principles which are beyond all worlds).

From this we see that matter can develop into life because life is already inherent in matter. Life can evolve mind, as mind is present in it as a seed. Just as milk can become butter by churning, so too are these different levels inherent in each other and can come out of each other by a process of growth. Nature is full of such capacity for transformation. This is the organic process of cosmic evolution.

THE THREE BODIES

According to Vedic science, the human being consists of three bodies. Through them and their indwelling consciousness we contain the entire universe and all its seven levels. Vedic cosmology is also Vedic psychology as all the universe is within us. Worlds exist only for the experience of the souls karmically tied to them.

The food and breath sheaths make up the gross or physical body, sthula sharira. The breath, emotion and intelligence sheaths make up the subtle or astral body, sukshma sharira. The intelligence and bliss sheaths make up the causal body, karana sharira.

Hence, between each body is an intermediate principle shared by both. Breath mediates between the astral and the physical. Intelligence, the power to ascertain truth and falsehood, mediates between the causal and the astral.

Bliss is also a dual principle and mediates between the causal body and the inner Self, whose nature is Being-Consciousness-Bliss, Sacchidananda.

The three bodies are the different vehicles of our consciousness. They are encasements for the inner being. Only the physical body is a body in our usual sense of the term. The astral has the same form as the physical body but is made up of subtle matter. The causal is of the form of an egg, a body of light.

Each of the three bodies relates to one of the three states of consciousness. The physical body is operative in the waking state, the astral body in dream and the causal body in deep sleep. The inner Self corresponds to the fourth state, turiya, the ever wakeful state of pure awareness. As we become more conscious, we also can become aware in the astral and causal bodies and learn to use their faculties as readily as those of the physical. However, many yogic teachings go directly to the inner Self and may not concern themselves with developing the potentials of these more subtle vehicles.

These three bodies correspond roughly to body, mind, and soul in the Western mystical traditions. The physical and astral bodies are formed anew at each incarnation. The causal body endures throughout the entire cycle of reincarnation and is the storehouse of all karmic impulses. It contains within itself the power to create the worlds, and through it we can be co-creators with God. At liberation it too is dissolved into its source consciousness.

THE SEVEN CHAKRAS

The seven chakras are the energy centers of the subtle body. They allow us experience of the different levels of the cosmos. Chakra itself means what revolves or a wheel. These centers have counterparts in the physical body. They are only truly awakened by Yogic practices, in which case they provide us with various occult or spiritual powers. In our ordinary state they do function, but on a reduced level. Chakra work or chakra balancing, as with the use of gems, sounds and colors, usually works on this outer level. It aids in the ordinary functioning of the chakras. Only our own practice of Yoga can really awaken the chakras into their inner power.

The Yoga of Knowledge usually does not deal with chakras at all. It goes directly to the pure Self which resides in the heart; not the heart center of the astral body but the spiritual heart on the right side of the body, which is behind the causal body and our point of contact with the universal consciousness transcending all the bodies.

The Yoga of Devotion also usually is not too concerned with the chakras. It emphasizes the heart chakra as the site of the Divine Beloved. Its main method is direct surrender to the Divine, not developing the intermediate powers.

The Yoga of Technique is most directly concerned with the chakras, though all systems of Yoga recognize their existence and their function. It has many practices for visualizing and energizing them, but even these are usually only done when these centers are in the process of naturally awakening, to help facilitate this process.

The Seven Chakras

1. Muladhara Chakra	The root center, literally the root foundation. It corresponds to the earth element and governs the systems of elimination, the survival instinct and the emotion of fear.
2. Svadhishthana Chakra	The sex center, literally the self-abode of the Kundalini. It corresponds to the element of water and governs the urino-genital systems, the sex instinct and the emotion of desire.
3. Manipura Chakra	The navel center, literally the city of gems. It corresponds to fire and governs the digestive system, the ego impulse and the emotion of anger.
4. Anahata Chakra	The heart center, literally the center of unstruck sound as from here emanates the subtle sounds (nada) of the subtle body. It relates to air, to the circulatory system, the individualized soul and the emotion of love.
5. Vishuddha Chakra	The throat center, literally the very pure. It relates to ether, the respiratory system, the higher intelligence and the power of communication.
6. Ajna Chakra	The third eye, literally the center of command. It relates to the mind generally and to the individual Self, to the power of inner perception.
7. Sahasrapadma Chakra	The head center, literally the thousand petalled lotus. It relates to the universal Self or Divine reality and to the power of consciousness itself.

THE NADIS

The Nadis are the nerves of the subtle body. They also connect us up with the subtle worlds, as we contain the entire universe within ourselves. Most important of the nadis are the solar and lunar nadis called the Pingala and the Ida. Between them runs the Sushumna, or central channel, on which the various chakras are strung like lotuses. It corresponds to the spinal canal of the physical body.

The solar nadi is of the nature of heat; the lunar of cold nature. Alternate nostril breathing is thereby used to balance the heat and cold and thereby regulate all metabolic processes in the body. Breathing in through the right and out through the left nostril increases heat in the body and dispels cold. Breathing in through the left and out through the right increases cold in the body and decreases heat.

For the awakening of the Kundalini, or power of consciousness, these two nadis must be purified and their energies balanced. This occurs naturally as consciousness evolves but can be hastened by the use of certain breathing or mantra practices.

10
DHARMIC PHILOSOPHIES
THEORIES OF TRUTH

Ever since late ancient times, the time of classical Greece, philosophy has been one of the greatest and most noble endeavors of the human mind. Human beings have struggled to create a true idea of the world or reality and to put into rational thought the order of the cosmos. Philosophical thinking has not been limited to the Western world. India has perhaps given birth to more different philosophies than any other country. Yet in India philosophy was primarily oriented to the spiritual life, to the practice of Yoga, and made subordinate to it. It was not considered an end in itself nor to be the highest aim of the mind. It is considered to be a stepping stone in training the mind. In the West, philosophy has been gradually subordinated to science and for this reason pure philosophy has declined and is largely disappearing. Yet, true philosophy, profound thinking and inquiry about the meaning of life, has always been one of the main ways of entering into the spiritual life. It is common to all people and all cultures though it may take a language other than that of reason.

The Vedas, the ancient scriptures of India, were written in a symbolic and mantric language. Hence, they do not set forth any definitive philosophy or world-view. They consist of the raw energy of spiritual experience prior to any systematization. They exist on an intuitive plane and come from a time when the intellect had yet to dominant human thought. Hence, they can be interpreted by the mind in many ways.

The later ancient scriptures of the Upanishads and the *Bhagavad Gita* also present a very wide and integral teaching. Any number of philosophical systems can be derived from them. None can claim to represent them solely. Even the Puranas and Tantras have many teachings on many different levels and a great deal of symbolism. Again, the emphasis is more on a broad teaching that gives individuals of different temperaments their own access to the truth rather than on setting forth any particular system.

Out of these broader teachings various more specific philosophies have arisen in time. Such philosophies and their differences of opinion are not always given much importance in the Yogic teaching, as it emphasizes direct perception and individual experience over textbook statements, even those of the greatest sages. Each individual has his own particular mind-set, as does each culture and each age. What is rational to one person or group may appear irrational to another. Hence, there can never be any ultimate philosophy everyone will agree upon. It is contrary to the nature of the mind and language itself, which tend toward differentiation. To insist upon such agreement is not helpful either, as it denies the creative unfoldment of the mind.

However, philosophies can be important for developing the rational powers of the mind and for attuning reason to the spiritual quest. They are a kind of mental exercise or gymnastic which can render the mind more fluid. The Indian philosophies also had their meditative practices to prove their main tenets. They cannot be understood on a purely conceptual or rational level without them. According to all the main philosophies of India, reason can organize but not cognize truth, for that, direct perception is required, which requires going beyond all mental preconceptions.

All the basic concepts for these philosophies can be found in ancient teachings like the *Rig Veda* in seed form, hidden in mantras, symbols, rituals and stories.

All the philosophies of India, including the non-orthodox Buddhist, Jain, and Sikh teachings share the following points:

> All hold that there exists a truth that is universal, infinite and eternal and it is the nature of consciousness itself.

> All hold that human beings are bound to a cycle of rebirth or reincarnation in ignorance of that truth. Our bondage is based upon ego and desire and results in suffering. It can only come to an end with the dissolution of ego and the renunciation of desire. Otherwise we will continue to be reborn until we have given up all desires.

> To this end of liberation we must follow the right values of truthfulness, non-violence, honesty, purity, simplicity.

> We must practice yoga and meditation to achieve this through silencing the mind. Various great sages who have achieved this state have left us teachings to follow which must be adapted by each individual.

Each of these teachings has its philosophical views. Not only do they refute the validity of each other's philosophy, they may refute the variant systems within their own tradition or religion. It was a style of debate in philosophy in medieval India to have to refute the validity of all views different from the philosopher's own and establish the sole rationality of his point of view.

We should also note that in these earlier times communication was not as good as it is today, so miscommunication was easier. Today, we find many of these arguments to be petty or merely semantic and are struck by the profound similarity and complementarity between these different systems of spiritual philosophy.

In this regard it should be remembered that all these teachings hold that truth transcends conceptual thought and can only be realized when we are free of all the biases, opinions and preconceptions of the mind. It appears that the holy wars which were fought in Europe and the Middle East on the battlefield were fought in the philosophical arena in more tolerant and more intellectual medieval India.

The orthodox or Vedic philosophies are six: 1) Sankhya, 2) Yoga, 3) Vedanta, 4) Mimamsa, 5) Nyaya, and 6) Vaisheshika. Each has its founder and its key text. Sankhya comes from the sage Kapila, though it is based on the *Sankhya Karika* of Ishwara Krishna (a different figure than Krishna of the *Gita*), as no works of Kapila remain. Yoga is based on the *Yoga Sutras* of Patanjali. Vedanta is based on the *Brahma Sutras* of Badarayana. Mimamsa is based upon the *Mimamsa Sutras* of Jaimini.

The prime texts or Sutras of these different systems are written in a very succinct language that rarely can be understood without a commentary. Hence, each of them has a primary commentary that is usually consulted. For example, Vyasa wrote the prime commentary on the *Yoga Sutras*. Shankara and Ramanuja wrote the main commentaries on the *Brahma Sutras*. These commentaries and some of the Sutras are usually much more recent than the original teachings, most of which were already in existence by the time of the Buddha. Nor is their any unanimous agreement on interpretation of these Sutras by their commentators. The different commentators may also disagree with or refute each other.

Sankhya and Yoga usually go together as Sankhya is the basic philosophy behind the classical yoga system. Vedanta and Mimamsa go together as Mimamsa is the ritual interpretation of the Vedas and Vedanta the knowledge or spiritual interpretation. Nyaya and Vaisheshika also go together as more mental or intellectual systems.

The main Buddhist philosophies are Sautrantika, Vijnanavada and Shunyavada. The Shunyavada system, based on the work of Nagarjuna, teaches the voidness of all reality. The Vijnanavada system, mainly of Vasubandhu, teaches the nature of reality as pure consciousness. The Sautrantika system teaches the momentary nature of all phenomenon.

A number of syncretic Hindu-Buddhist teachings arose, combining both together. This occurred more commonly in Indonesia and Indochina in medieval times, perhaps also in central Asia. It still occurs in Nepal today, where both Hindu and Buddhist deities and yogis are worshipped together. However, no unified Hindu-Buddhist philosophical teachings remain, though some have attempted this in modern times.

SANKHYA

The most basic philosophy of India is the Sankhya system. All the other philosophies orthodox and unorthodox show much influence from it. Though they may disagree with it as to ultimate principles, they follow its structure and logic. Sankhya goes back to Kapila, who is mentioned as early as the *Rig Veda.* Kapila was for centuries the most famous sage in India. His fame rivaled that of Krishna or Buddha and was not eclipsed until the time of Shankara (c. 600 A.D.). His name was synonymous with wisdom itself. Most of the Sankhya teachings, however, have been lost in time, except for some later philosophical texts.

At the time of Krishna and in the *Bhagavad Gita,* Sankhya, Yoga and Vedanta were one, and he taught all three as aspects of the same truth. It was only in the philosophical era which began after the time of the Buddha that these teachings split into opposing camps, usually over minor conceptual differences. They all share the same basic system and terminology and look back to the Vedas and Upanishads for their inspiration and authorization.

Sankhya means literally the science of enumeration. It lists the basic principles of the cosmic existence. These are twenty-four. They are: 1) prime matter (Prakriti); 2) cosmic mind (Mahat); 3) ego (ahamkara); 4) mind (manas); 5-9) the five tanmatras, or prime qualities, or root principles of sound, touch, sight, taste and hearing; 10-14) the five sense organs: ear, skin, eye, tongue, and nose; 15-19) the five organs of action: mouth, hands, feet, sexual organ, and anus; and 20-24) the five gross elements of ether, air, fire, water and earth.

Purusha or Pure Consciousness may be listed among these as the first, but strictly speaking it is outside of manifestation.

All the other systems have similar lists of principles based upon the organs and elements (called aggregates or skandhas in Buddhist thought). Some Tantric systems expand this list to 36.

Sankhya teaches that there are two ultimate principles: the principle of consciousness or the seer, called the Purusha, and the principle of appearance or the seen, called Prakriti. Purusha is the ground of consciousness. Prakriti is the essential stuff of experience. The purpose of yoga is to move from identification with the seen back into the pure consciousness of the seer, which is ever free, blissful and infinite.

THE THREE GUNAS

Prakriti, Primal Nature, is said to consist of three qualities, called gunas or ropes, as they are the factors of bondage. These are the principle of light and lightness, called sattva, meaning goodness or virtue; rajas, the principle of energy or turbulence, literally referring to the storm; and tamas, the principle of inertia and heaviness.

Tamas is black and relates to the Earth and the night in the Vedic system. Rajas is red and relates to the Atmosphere and the Dawn. Sattva is white and corresponds to Heaven and the Day.

All objects in nature are combinations of these three gunas. From them evolve all the other qualities we see in things, like hardness, softness, heaviness, lightness, heat and cold, etc. All objects are nothing but collections of qualities. Hence, there is no real object in itself other than consciousness. If we take the roof, floor and walls from a house, what house is left over? It is only an experience in the mind.

Sattva is the natural quality of the mind, rajas of the life-force and tamas of the physical body. When rajas and tamas occur in the mind, they become the factors of ignorance and dullness (tamas) and distraction and desire (rajas). All Yoga consists of reducing rajas and tamas from the mind to bring it to a state of pure sattva. Pure sattva, or the mind in its natural state, has the power to perceive the truth, to reflect the seer or the Purusha.

The three gunas give us a system of understanding the quality or spiritual value in things. They are used for classifying all the things of our life: our food, thoughts, emotions, impressions, our beliefs and aspirations.

Hence, the Yogic diet always aims at taking predominately sattvic food, living in a sattvic environment, associating with sattvic people and having a generally sattvic life-style. Sattvic food is vegetarian, fresh, organic and prepared with love. A sattvic environment is natural, pure, quiet, and harmonious. Sattvic people are possessed of love, faith, devotion, honesty and truthfulness.

YOGA

The system of Yoga takes over the entire philosophy of Sankhya. It adds Ishwara, the personal God, as an additional principle. Yet for it Ishwara is not the creator of the world so much as the Divine teacher or Cosmic guru. Sankhya philosophy recognizes a kind of demiurge or cosmic lord but emphasizes the pure consciousness beyond all manifestation as the true Divine.

Yoga adds its practical system of development, its eight limbs (ashtanga) to the Sankhya system. These are right attitudes (yama), right observances (niyama), yogic postures (asana), breath-control (pranayama), control of the senses (pratyahara), attention (dharana), meditation (dhyana) and absorption (samadhi). They are practical, not philosophical, principles and are used by all the systems.

VEDANTA

Vedanta recognizes a cosmic Lord or Ishwara as the creator, sustainer and destroyer of the universe. Many Vedantic systems also consider Prakriti, primal Nature, to be Maya, a power of illusion which is ultimately unreal. The systems that teach Maya as illusion are non-dualist (advaita); they say that reality is One only, even God being ultimately unreal. There are also realistic forms of non-duality which see all things as manifestations of the One truth.

Dualistic systems of Vedanta exist as well, being primarily theistic in nature. Yet, even these accept non-duality as one aspect of truth. In this regard they are much more complex and sophisticated than the dualistic systems of Judeao-Christian and Islamic religions, which do not usually allow for any experience of monism or the identity of the individual soul with the transcendent Divine.

Basic Vedantic Concepts

Atman	The inner or higher Self. There is the individual self (jivatman) and the supreme or absolute Self (paramatman). The two in essence are one just as the universal space is one with the space enclosed within a jar.
Brahman	The absolute or supreme reality, the unborn, uncreate transcendent existence.
Ishvara	The personal God or the power of Brahman in creation.

BUDDHIST SYSTEMS

Buddhist philosophy rejects any Ishwara or Cosmic Lord. The Mahayana philosophies, those of the great vehicle, also regard Nature as Maya or illusion, or as the Void. They teach non-dualism as well, so they are the Buddhist counterpart of the Mayavada, the Advaita Vedanta teaching. However, these Buddhist systems do not regard pure consciousness as Atma, the inner Self, but see it as devoid of any sense of self. Some Buddhist systems, like the Vijnanavada, use such terms as Prajnatman, or the Self of wisdom, and thereby come closer to the Vedantic view.

JAINISM

The Jains emphasize a path of action. As such, they did not develop philosophy to a high degree, though they did have their philosophies. They considered it of more importance to learn through action rather than through speculative thought.

SYNTHESIS

While these philosophies differ as to details, each represents an important truth or insight also recognized by the others. These can be summarized as follows:

Sankhya	Its fundamental insight is the discrimination between Spirit and matter, the inner and the outer, consciousness and form. This is the starting point of all spiritual teachings. It also presents an ordering of cosmic principles according to the faculties of our nature and our capacity for experience on different levels. This examination of the process of perception and the nature of consciousness is followed by all systems.
Yoga	Its fundamental insight is the need for practise and its outline of the eightfold or integral Yoga path. All these systems use some form of Yoga and resort to some form of each of its eight limbs. All have their attitudes and values, use Yoga postures, examine the breath, and teach meditation.
Vedanta	Its fundamental insight is the sole reality of the Self or the inner consciousness and the unreality of all we think is other than it. It also stresses the truth of the absolute unity of all life. Dualistic Vedanta emphasizes devotion and the need for the worship of the Divine.
Mimamsa	Its fundamental insight is the need for rituals in our outer life to help attune ourselves and our society to the ritual order of the cosmos. All systems employ such rituals to enhance or protect their teaching.
Sautrantika	Its fundamental insight is the transient and momentary nature of all things. The spiritual life is always a movement from the transient to the eternal.

Vijnanavada	Its fundamental insight is that reality consists of pure consciousness. While the different systems may define consciousness differently, all agree that it is ultimately indefinable.
Shunyavada	Its fundamental insight is that truth transcends all the concepts of the mind. Vedanta also accepts this, as do Sankhya and Yoga. It is the neti-neti doctrine, the great negation taught in the Upanishads

PHILOSOPHY IN THE NEW AGE

We see that there is nothing in these systems which is necessarily contradictory to the others, unless we are overly insistent upon the semantics of the presentation. Today, we are living in an age of synthesis and reconciliation. We are no longer aiming at sharpening the intellect but increasing its grasp and moving beyond it. From this perspective, philosophy must take on a new orientation. The philosophical age is over. What we need today is a new age of practical experimentation in the spiritual realm based upon an attitude of openness, freedom and a non-insistence upon any names or forms of the mind.

The mind in its active mode is not the instrument of spiritual knowledge. Truth perception requires passivity of the mind. It is this which we must give priority to. While spiritual philosophies can help train our minds and give us an idea of what is to be accomplished, we must be willing to set them aside, to go to the real truth which no words can ever describe or delimit, positively or negatively.

11
THE PATHS
OF YOGA

Seers of the vast illumined seer yogically control their
intelligence and mind. The One knower of all the ways
of wisdom, he ordains the invocations of the Gods.
Great is the affirmative being of the Divine solar Will.
                                        — Rig Veda, V. 81. 1.

YOGA

In the Vedic teaching it is not enough merely to learn something
theoretically or conceptually. The intellect is not the instrument of real
knowledge. Whatever we learn must be put into practice in our daily life,
with body, speech, mind and full awareness. It is only when it becomes
part of our nature, when through it we change who we are and thereby
return to our higher nature, that it can be said to be really known or
accomplished. This practical application of the Vedic teaching is called
Yoga. As practice is more important than theory, Yoga is more important
than Veda, though neither should be separated from the other.

The term Yoga itself means to combine, coordinate, harmonize,
integrate, utilize. It indicates the maximum coordination of energy towards transformation or liberation. All these meanings are present in the
basic root of yoga, 'yuj'. This, in turn, is based on a more simple root 'yu'.
'Yu' evolves from the vowel sound 'i' meaning will, direction, velocity,
command, or concentration. 'Yu' itself means both to unite or to separate,
to unite with the real and separate from the unreal. To it is combined the
consonant 'j' additionally emphasizing energy, creativity and direction.
Hence, the meaning of Yoga arises as integration, discrimination and
discipline. There are many synonyms for Yoga in Sanskrit and other
languages. It is often called the way or the path or the work.

Yoga, as work, is not our ordinary work of seeking to gain things for
ourselves or become something. It is not some form of attainment,
achievement or acquisition. It is the spiritual work of dissolving our
egoistic drives into the cosmic will. As such, it is a path of inaction or
action opposite the ordinary direction of outward expansion. It involves
meditation, patience, perseverance, silence, solitude and peace. The anal-

ogy of Yoga is like making an irrigation ditch from a river to irrigate a piece of land. The work does not create the water but only makes a channel for it to flow. Without contact with the inner waters of truth, Yoga therefore has no purpose. Hence, in the ancient writings Yoga was also called 'Yajna', meaning sacrifice, surrender, offering or consecration. The Yogic work is the sacrifice of the outer and the lower to afford a path for the inner and the higher to manifest.

Yoga proceeds by a special grace or power. This is called the Yoga Shakti, or power of Yoga. It is the Yoga Shakti that does the real work, not our personal will. This Yoga Shakti is the inner form of the Goddess, the secret energy and intelligence of Mother Nature in evolution. It is the natural intelligence of the Yoga Shakti, which is the power of nature herself, that directs and plans the work of Yoga, not our own personal mentality. We can aid in her work. By our assent to the work we allow her force to act within us. But we cannot do the work ourselves. What is mortal, finite and limited cannot become immortal, infinite or unlimited. But if we surrender our mortal nature to a higher aspiration, we can create the space, the field and the matrix for the immortal powers to manifest themselves.

There are many different paths and styles of Yoga but all come under five different areas:

1) The Path of Knowledge, 2) The Path of Devotion, 3) The Path of Technique, 4) The Path of Service, and 5) The Integral Path combining all four.

While all spiritual and religious teachings have their practice, their Yoga, it is in the Eternal Teaching or Sanatana Dharma from the Himalayas that we find the greatest diversity and freedom of such approaches. It has no insistence that the individual must follow one path or another. Even within a particular path there is no insistence that the individual must follow one approach or another. What is essential is that we follow a path, one which most appeals to our inner nature and true heart, and that we give our full attention and dedication to it, not as a matter of personal effort or striving, but as the expression of the fullness of our life and being and our need to transcend. As usual in the systems of Vedic knowledge, the attitude and concentration is what matters, not the form.

The classical Yoga system of India is the Raja Yoga system outlined in the *Yoga Sutras* of Patanjali, which appear to date around the third century B.C. The term Yoga however is found already in the *Bhagavad Gita* and the Upanishads and is present in some very important Vedic hymns also, both in the *Rig* and *Yajur Vedas*. Most commonly the term Yajna, sacrifice, as already indicated, is used in the Vedas instead of Yoga.

The most significant ancient form of Yoga was Mantra Yoga, or the Yoga of the Divine Word. This Yoga is hidden in all the scriptures of the ancient world. Hence, Yoga is as old as man and as old as human language. Language itself arose at first as an effort to communicate with God and his cosmic powers and presence, as a means of reintegration of the human with the universal.

Life itself is Yoga; that is, there is an ongoing will in life towards growth, evolution and transformation. This will towards Yoga inherent in life is the Vedic Sun God of inspiration, Savitar, who is behind the manifestation of all the Gods. Life is also Yoga in the sense that it is an ongoing work producing a specific result. Whatever we do is a kind of Yoga, a concerted action to gain a particular end. While normally we unconsciously practice Yoga, making various efforts to develop our outer powers to gain the outer aims of life, in Yoga itself we learn to consciously direct our energies to gain the inner aim of liberation. For this Yoga shows us how to align ourselves with the cosmic intelligence and use the cosmic energy. This provides a much greater power of action and transformation than the normal usage of our personal energies. The Yogic path we follow should reflect what really attunes us to this greater Divine force.

THE YOGA OF KNOWLEDGE
Jnana Yoga

In the Vedic system knowledge is defined as both higher and lower or superior and inferior (para and apara). The lower or inferior knowledge consists of the knowledge of the outer world. It consists of name and form and is concerned with the measurable. Through it we can recognize the objects of the world and learn how to use them. All science is a form of the lower knowledge, as it is based on measurement and mathematics and the information which comes to us through the senses. Take away the measurable and what is left of science? Remove our names and what do we really know about things?

We see that this form of knowledge is limited and superficial. It gives us a way of manipulating external things, but it does not give us a sense of their intrinsic being. For example, science can tell us about the chemical composition of a star, but what is its being, its soul, its purpose in creation? That is beyond the scope of science to judge. The lower knowledge has its place. It helps us deal with the outer aspects of life, but it is insufficient for knowledge of absolute truth or reality. This is common knowledge to many scientists also, who see the inherent limitations of their approach.

Even the conceptual or theoretical knowledge of spiritual teachings is a form of outer knowledge. All second hand knowledge is outer knowledge. It is all limited and consists ultimately only of words and memory patterns which have no power to change what is.

We are reminded of the soliloquy of Faust who lists his mastery of all forms of knowledge and his lack of any true certainty, peace or happiness through them. In the Upanishads, Narada approaches Sanat Kumara, the eternal child (innocent mind) and World teacher. Sanat Kumara asks him what he knows. He lists all the Vedas, all the arts and sciences of his day, from astrology to archery. Sanat Kumara states that all this knowledge is only a name. To go beyond sorrow we must know ourselves. The outer knowledge, however fascinating, however much control of the external it gives, cannot give understanding of who we really are. Hence, it can create more outer energy than we have the inner wisdom to deal with, which is root of the present crisis in humanity.

The higher knowledge is concerned with knowledge of the immeasurable, nameless, formless and absolute reality. It has no specific conceptual content. It is not a matter of theory or information. It is the knowledge of consciousness itself. Whereas the lower knowledge is based on the observation of external things, the objects presented to us via the senses, the higher knowledge is based on self-observation. Whereas the lower knowledge works through the mind as its vehicle and accepts the basic patterns of the mind, the higher knowledge is based on observation of the mind itself and seeing its inherent limitations. The lower knowledge proceeds through the activity of the mind, whereas the higher knowledge comes through its passivity.

The mind must always think in terms of time, place, cause and effect. These are its a priori categories. They are not philosophical principles but the inherent structure of the mind whose focus is outward directed. The mind is based on thought, which is name, form and person (self-image). Observing the mind, we gain the capacity to go beyond its structure and its inherent limitation. We become free of attachment and limitation to time, place and person and come gradually to know the eternal, infinite and absolute. To look at things through the mind is to become caught in an idea, judgement or opinion about them. To examine things directly is to find the one in all and all in one. Even modern science is discovering that these basic constructs of the mind of time and space do not reflect the truth of things or the foundation of the universe.

Liberation, the goal of the Yoga of knowledge, is defined as the discrimination between the thoughts of the mind and the consciousness of the observer, or state of seeing which is beyond thought. The Yoga of Knowledge, Jnana Yoga, has usually been considered to be the highest and ultimate of the Yogic paths. The classical definition of Yoga by

Patanjali is the "silencing of the thought patterns of the mind" (citta vrtti nirodha, *Yoga Sutras I. 2.*). This is the definition of knowledge or wisdom.

***

The Yoga of knowledge is not a matter of acquiring theoretical or practical information. It is not the practice of the thinking mind, though it may start out with deep pondering of the primary questions of life (such as "who am I," or "what is God, Truth or Reality?"). It is the practice of meditation, which is the mind in the state of non-judgmental observation. Hence, the classical Jnani, or man of spiritual knowledge, is quite different than the philosopher straining at subtle ideas. He is often silent, impersonal and inactive, like the natural sage of Lao-Tse. Yogic knowledge is the state of awareness itself, which has no object and seeks no end, which relies on no book but reads the message of life moment by moment.

Hence, there is little theory to the Yoga of knowledge. Its prime statement is simple — Know Thyself. It usually avoids all metaphysical theories and discussions, including how did the world begin or what is the order of creation. Some knowledge teachings do not even require belief in God, guru, or any religious faith and are outside of any formality or ceremony. They state that all explanations of things belong to the mind. The truth is something that cannot be put into words, which is beyond all theories, outside of all beliefs. It has to be experienced in the state of seeing, which can only be learned through choiceless observation. Hence, Jnana Yoga is very simple, though very hard to do, as it requires going beyond our very mind and habitual thought process.

Self-Inquiry

The most basic practise of the Yoga of knowledge is Self-inquiry (Atma vichara). It consists of tracing the self or "I" thought to its origin. If we observe our minds carefully, we see that all thoughts are based upon the "I-thought." We cannot think about anything without first having an idea about ourselves. But if we look deeply, we see that the "I" itself is something unknown to us.

We are constantly projecting our identity on some external object or quality: "I am this, this is mine." We are constantly mixing this unknown "I" without some known thing. "I am good or bad; I am wise or foolish; I am happy or sad; I am a Hindu, Buddhist or Christian; I am an American or Russian; I am black or white or yellow." All of these are thoughts in which the "I" is referred to an object that is really different from it. What the "I" is in itself we do not know and cannot know as long as we are projecting it on to something.

Our most basic projection is our self-image, which is our "I am the body" idea. Yet, we can observe our body grow and decline. We can perceive it as an instrument or vehicle we use but as different from who we really are. If we are perceptive, we can discern that our basic consciousness or state of seeing is ever pure, beyond all external changes. Though our body may age and our thoughts may change, our seeing is eternal. As long as we are identified with the body, or through it with any external thing, we must suffer, because all external things are transient and we long for eternal and permanent happiness. Our very longing for this lasting happiness is proof of our nature in consciousness as blissful and pure.

This does not mean that the body is bad or sinful or to be denied. It is the best vehicle nature can provide. Yet it is only a vehicle. It is no more who we are than our car is. In no longer identifying with the body, we come to treat it properly and no longer abuse it for personal gratification.

Teachings on the Yoga of Knowledge

Many knowledge teachings exist. Most classically from India is the Vedantic path. This is embodied in the Upanishads (particularly the *Kena*) and the *Bhagavad Gita*. The Sankhya and Yoga teachings as in the *Yoga Sutras* are also primarily versions of the Yoga of Knowledge. The Yoga of Knowledge is most specifically related in the works of Advaita Vedanta, like the *Ashtavakra Samhita* or *Avadhut Gita*. On a more scholarly level it is represented by the works of Shankara and his followers and the school of Advaita Vedanta. Other great schools of knowledge are Kashmiri Shaivism, South India Shaiva Siddhanta, etc.

The Yoga of knowledge is very prominent in the Buddhist tradition, wherein it is usually more emphasized than the other yogas. Such practices as Tibetan Mahamudra and Dzog Chen, Chinese Chan and Japanese Zen, and the southern Vipassana traditions are essentially versions of the Yoga of knowledge passed on from India through Buddhist sources.

There are many modern teachers including Ramana Maharshi, Swami Vivekananda and Swami Rama Tirtha for Vedanta. J. Krishnamurti also gives a very pure and modern Yoga of knowledge approach, free of all traditional and cultural forms.

THE YOGA OF DEVOTION
Bhakti Yoga

Love is the basis of all life. Without it we cannot live. God is often defined as love. Most of our lives are spent seeking love. But what is love, do we really know? Is our seeking based on truth or illusion? Will it bring us to true love or some form of disappointment or dissipation?

Love, like knowledge, can be distinguished as higher and lower. The lower form of love is sexual passion or any need to attach ourselves to external things. It is the need to be loved. The higher form of love is devotion, love of God, love of Truth, love of Life. It is the willingness to give love. In the lower form of love we seek love from the outside, from someone or some body. In the higher form of love we go to the source of love within and are willing to be a source of that love for all. We must seek love as love is our nature, but it is up to us whether it is the higher or lower form we align ourselves with.

Devotion or Divine love is the second major path of Yoga. It consists of the worship of the Divine Beloved. This can be through various chosen deities (Ishta devatas) or incarnations of God (Avatars). Sometimes the teacher or guru may become the object of worship. This does not mean to worship their outer personality but to give reverence to the Divine teacher within them.

A personal form of the Divine is often used as an aid in devotion. After all, we naturally project our devotion on a form or personality, that being our human condition for many life-times. But the form is a means to the formless, a symbol to aid in the concentration of the mind. As we move along the path of devotion, we begin to find the Beloved, our form of the Divine, everywhere and in all things. We move from the outer form of the Divine, the person, to the inner form which is the Word, to the true nature which is Being itself. Eventually, we must come to realize our Beloved as the Divine presence in our own hearts, our own inner or true Self.

Devotional practices consist of rituals (puja), singing (kirtan), chanting names of God (japa), and meditation on a form of the Divine (upasana).

Women may worship the Divine in the male form like Shiva, Krishna or Rama. Men may worship the Divine in a female form as the different aspects of the Goddess (Devi). This reflects our natural impulse to find our opposite in love. Such deities become the muse or inner guide along the path. Yet we may also worship the Divine in a kindred form; the ascetic yogi worshipping Shiva or the female yogini worshipping the form of the Divine Mother she seeks to incarnate. Every variation is possible and each has its beauty and purpose in creation.

India has always taught freedom of worship. This is the real reason for the great variety of Gods and Goddesses in the teaching. It is not some primitive polytheism, though less developed souls may use it in this way, but a great creative openness which provides a form of the Divine approach for each individual. The Sanatana Dharma, or eternal religion, as already mentioned, holds that ultimately each individual must have his or her own religion. We should each create our own Gods and scriptures. Ultimately, the entire universe is our creation.

Each one of us is entitled to worship the Divine in whatever form our heart seeks. Let be a stone, a tree, a cloud or let be Christ or Krishna, male or female, the most noble ideal or great concept, that is not the issue. What is important is that we really give our hearts to the Divine. The form is an aid and a catalyst and in the end must be dissolved into the universal Godhead.

Bhakti Yoga is often related to Karma Yoga, as it usually involves either service to the Divine or service to humanity. While devotion is the proper attitude of the soul towards the Divine, compassion is the proper attitude of the Divine and the awakened soul towards the rest of creation. True compassion is a Divine quality and can only come from an inner connection with the Divine. It is not to be confused with pity that looks down on others. It is a force of unity which respects the Divine power and intelligence in each and seeks to aid in its unfoldment.

Christianity itself is primarily a teaching of the Yoga of Devotion. All the practices of the Yoga of Devotion can be adapted to Christ, the Madonna or to the various saints of the Christian tradition. Islam itself is primarily devotional, but it follows a strict formless devotion which prohibits all use of images, though the *Koran,* like the *Bible,* uses many poetic metaphors, the images of the mind. Hinduism contains a similar devotional approach, but is wider in scope and linked to all the other Yoga paths.

Devotion also appeals to an artistic mentality. The muse is nothing but a lower form of the Divine beloved. The use of images, statues, rituals and chants is a subtle form of art and poetry directed towards the Divine through devotion. Art is in its true form a path of devotion. It directs the mind and the senses towards the appreciation of the eternal.

Great modern teachers of the Yoga of Devotion include Ramakrishna, Paramahansa Yogananda, Anandamayi Ma, Sri Aurobindo and the Mother. The list could be made much longer, as devotion is perhaps the essence of Hinduism. The classical text is Narada's *Bhakti Sutras.* Philosophies have been built on devotion also like the Vedantic approaches of Ramanuja and Madhva. These express theism as the ultimate reality and give emphasis to the personality of the Divine. But they recognize the unity of the Godhead as the basis of the play of the Divine personality.

FORMS OF THE GODS AND GODDESSES

The five main deities in India are Shiva, Vishnu, the Devi, Ganesh and Surya. As Ganesh, the elephant faced God, is the son of Shiva his worship is often included under that of Shiva. As Surya, the Sun, is generally a form of Vishnu, his worship can be included under his. In medieval India the Buddha was the sixth form of worship. Each God has his consort or Goddess, like Vishnu and Lakshmi, but the Goddess is also worshipped in her own right. Her main form is the consort of Shiva, and in this regard she has many names and forms like Kali, Durga, Parvati, Uma, Sati, Maheshwari, etc. While the main forms and practices of devotional worship are the same for all deities, each has its particular approaches.

THE TRINITY

The Hindu trinity is of Brahma, Vishnu and Shiva. They are respectively the creator, preserver and destroyer of the universe. They are also aligned as the transcendent Godhead, Shiva, the cosmic lord, Vishnu, and the cosmic mind, Brahma. In this regard they are called Sat-Tat-Aum, the Being, the Thatness or immanence and the Word or holy spirit. This is much like the Christian trinity of God as the Father, Son and Holy Ghost. The trinity represents the Divine in its threefold nature and function. Each aspect of the trinity contains and includes the others.

Each God in the trinity has his consort. For Brahma is Saraswati, the Goddess of knowledge. For Vishnu is Lakshmi, the Goddess of love, beauty and delight. For Shiva is Kali, the Goddess of power, destruction and transformation. These are the three main forms of the Goddess, as Brahma, Vishnu and Shiva are the three main forms of the God. The three Goddesses are often worshipped in their own right as well as along with their spouses.

GODS
Shiva

Shiva is the great God, Mahadeva. He represents the pure existence or Divine will beyond creation. He is, therefore, the lord of Yogis and the lord of Jnanis, those who pursue the Yoga of Knowledge.

Shiva has many names, like Shankara, Shambhu, Sadashiva, Rudra, Bhava, Sharva, Pashupati, Aghora, and Bhairava. Shiva itself means the beneficent or auspicious. Some of his forms, like Shiva and Shankara, are beneficent. Others, like Rudra and Bhairava, are terrible. The terrible forms are useful for removing any negativity from our spiritual lives. They become our protectors.

In Nepal, Indonesia, and Indochina a cult of Shiva-Buddha arose, combining the qualities of these two related great religious forms.

Nataraj

One of his main forms is Shiva Nataraja, Shiva as the Lord of the cosmic dance. He performs the mighty tandava, the dance of destruction that destroys the universe. This is also the dance of knowledge that takes us from the unreal to the real, from the ignorance to the knowledge, from the ego to the Self.

Ganesh

Ganesh, the elephant God, is the first son of Shiva and Parvati. He is a God of both wisdom and wealth. He removes all obstructions and grants us the fruit of our actions. Hence, he is invoked before any major project in life. His temples are quite numerous, particularly in the south of India.

Ganesh is a very Kapha (watery) God and is full of love and joy. He holds the entire universe in his belly. He is a little like the laughing Buddha in Chinese imagery. He can also be found in Buddhist and Jain temples and is one of the most widely revered of all the Gods. Ganesh is also called Ganapati. Both names mean the lord of hosts as he rules the whole group of the Gods.

Skanda

Skanda is the second son of Shiva and Parvati. He is the war God, the Hindu equivalent of Mars and Ares. He was created to lead the heavenly hosts and destroy the demons. He is the most masculine and fierce of all the Gods. He is also fire, Agni, and is very Pitta (fiery) in nature. While Ganesh removes all obstacles, Skanda bestows all spiritual powers, particularly the power of knowledge.

His other names are Karttikeya, Guha, and Shadannana or Shanmukha (as he has six faces). He is also called Sanat Kumara, the eternal child.

Vishnu

Vishnu is Narayana, the Cosmic Man or the Divine being who has entered into mortals. He is also Surya or Savitar, the Sun or the solar logos. He is the Divine presence which pervades all creation. Vishnu literally means the Pervader, as he is the immanent divine consciousness that gives order to the worlds, which by its three steps measures creation.

The Avatars

The Puranas recognize ten avatars. All avatars come from Vishnu, as he is the indwelling guiding cosmic lord and intelligence. He is the cosmic guru.

These avatars are the fish (matsya), turtle (kurma), boar (varaha), manlion (nrisimha), dwarf (vamana), Parashurama, Rama, Krishna, Buddha and Kalki. Parashurama shows the man of power; Rama, the Divine warrior and protector; Krishna, the Divine lover; Buddha, the Divine sage; and Kalki, the completer and saviour. In this scheme we see the idea of the evolution of the soul from the animal realms to perfect spiritual knowledge.

The idea of the messiah came to the Western religions of Judaism, Christianity and Islam from the Zoroastrian religion of ancient Persia. Zoroastrianism has ten incarnations of Vrithragna (Indra). Hence, it is related to the avatar idea of the Hindus.

Rama

Ram is one of the great Gods of the ancient world. We find him in India, in both Hindu and Buddhist annals. He was said to have brought the Aryan dharma to the south of India and out to sea. He was also worshipped in Indonesia and Indochina. He is related to Amon Re (Om Ram) of the Egyptians, as a form of the Sun God, particularly the night Sun that destroys the demons and takes us across the ocean of darkness.

Sita, his consort, is the Earth Goddess. She is the receptive mind, the power of pure devotion. When we lose our Sita, we lose everything because we lose the humility which allows us to grow. In the *Ramayana* she is stolen from Rama by the demon, Ravana, who took the form of a Brahmin to deceive her.

Rama's main helper is Hanuman or Maruti, the Monkey God, a form of the Wind God. Rama, Hanuman and Sita thus represent the Sun, the wind and the Earth or the three worlds of the Vedas and their respective powers.

Rama also was an historical figure as well as a mythic image. He was said to have reigned in north India in Ayodhya in the latter part of the Silver Age or Treta Yuga (c. 4000 B.C.).

Krishna

Krishna is the foremost of the avatars, the personification of Divine love and delight. We find the figure of the Divine player of the flute all over the world. It is a common image in Sufi poetry and can be found in Europe and in ancient America as well, one of the main archetypes of the Divine in the human mind.

Yet Krishna was an actual historical figure as well. He was born in Mathura (south of Delhi) and reigned later at Dwaraka in Gujarat. He died at the age of 125.

There are many forms of Krishna also. There is the baby Krishna, the boy Krishna, Krishna the young lover, Krishna the warrior, Krishna the king, and Krishna the sage.

Krishna's two main consorts are Radha and Rukmini, the former his young beloved, the latter his queen. He had many other consorts as well, the Gopis, for each of whom he assumed a separate form. Actually, all souls are consorts of Krishna who is the Divine lover.

Buddha

Buddha was introduced into the scheme of avatars at a later period as part of an attempt to integrate Hinduism and Buddhism. His own teachings were not studied or included among the literature on the avatars, though the stories of the Buddha follow a similar epic style as the *Puranas*. He is a major archetypal figure in the human mind and has become the human type who most represents Indian spirituality to the world, the sage in meditation.

Kalki

Kalki is the Hindu Messiah. He will come at the end of the dark age to destroy the wicked and restore the rule of truth on the Earth. According to some, he has already taken birth and will usher in a new spiritual age for humanity. Certainly, his energy is quite needed today. His vehicle is a white horse. He is not as commonly mentioned as Rama or Krishna.

GODDESSES
Saraswati
Vak

Saraswati is worshipped along with any study or learning. Chants to her often begin and end classes on Vedic studies. She is the Goddess of the Word. She is purity itself and always wears white. She holds a vina, a book and a rosary. Her sacred syllable is Aim. She represents the stream of wisdom, the free flow of the knowledge of consciousness.

She is the form of the Goddess most mentioned in the Vedas, as she is Vedamata, the mother of the Vedas, the mother of knowledge. She also appears in Buddhist iconography as the consort of Manjushri, the God of wisdom.

Ganga

All rivers are forms of the Goddess. They represent the river of knowledge. Ganga, the Goddess of the Ganges river, is much like Saraswati. After the Saraswati river went dry in ancient times, much of the reverence attached to it was transferred to the Ganges as the center of the culture shifted slightly to the east.

Lakshmi
Shri

Lakshmi is the most commonly worshipped of the Goddesses, and images of her can be found throughout India. She is still widely worshipped, even among the Muslims in Indonesia as Dewi Shri. She is the Goddess of wealth, good fortune, good luck, beauty and fertility. As these are the main objects of our seeking in life, naturally this form of the Goddess has always had the main attraction for the human mind.

She has a higher form, however, as Divine love and beauty, the power of devotion. Her mantra is Shrim (shreem).

Parvati
Uma

The Goddess as the wife of Shiva is known as Parvati, the Goddess of the mountain or of the mountain stream. She is also called Girija, the mountain born. She is the pure consciousness born in the mountains of meditation, the mystic Himalayas. She is the form of the power of consciousness.

As the giver of knowledge, she is known as Uma, the protectress. As the pure being, consecrated in the fire of knowledge, she is known as Sati.

Kali

Kali is the Goddess of death and transformation. She has a ghostly appearance, a dark or black color. She arises from the chest of Shiva (a corpse). She is the main terrible form of the Goddess. Through her we break through all attachments and go beyond all the illusions and sufferings of the world. She is the love that endures beyond death and which thereby takes us beyond death. Her mantra is Klim (kleem).

Durga

Durga is the Goddess as the demon-slayer. She rides a lion. Her nature is also very fiery (Pitta). She destroys all negativity and illusion. Another name for her is Chamunda, the fierce one. She saves us and delivers us across all the difficulties of life. Hence, in all dangers she is to be invoked. Her mantra is Dum (doom).

Lalita
Tripurasundari

Shiva's consort is not only a Goddess of power and death, she is also a Goddess of beauty and delight. As Tripurasundari, the beauty of the three worlds, she represents the beauty of the natural world, all the universe in the glory of God or pure consciousness. As Lalita, the delightful one, she is the bliss that comes to us through knowledge. The thousand names of Lalita are one of the main forms of worship of the Goddess. Her mantra is Hrim (hreem).

Tara

Tara is an important Hindu Goddess, as well as the main Buddhist Goddess. In Hinduism she is related to Durga as the power which takes us across (tarati) all danger and darkness. In the Buddhist system she is Wisdom, the Mother of the Buddhas, which delivers us across ignorance. She has many forms as white, green, etc. She is commonly worshipped in Tibet and under the form of Kwan Yin in China.

Some scholars have tried to divide off the Buddhist from the Hindu Goddesses saying the former represent wisdom (prajna) and the latter represent power (shakti). However, we see in the Vedic system that the Goddesses have three aspects, wisdom (Saraswati), love (Lakshmi) and power (Kali). These three always go together and do not exclude each other. True power is through wisdom which is love. Hence, the power we see worshipped in the Hindu Goddesses is always the power of consciousness or wisdom (Chit-Shakti).

THE YOGA OF SERVICE
Karma Yoga

All spiritual teachings speak of our need to help the world and to uplift humanity. Hence, most practitioners of Yoga are expected to do some work of service, Sanskrit seva, to humanity. This may be providing food or clothing to the poor or needy, working in schools or hospitals, or distributing books and teachings.

There are very few books on Karma Yoga, nor does it have its special Sutras or texts like the other Yoga paths. Yet it is given its importance in all approaches, particularly the Yoga of Devotion. Mahatma Gandhi was a good modern representative of this approach.

Generally speaking, the Yogic teaching, as it is non-political and inward oriented, does not emphasize service and charity as much as Christianity. Moreover, unlike many so-called Christian groups, it does not consider it to be true service to others to try to convert them to our beliefs. True service is in helping others to help themselves, aiding them in unburdening themselves, not imposing new ideas upon them. To provide food, shelter or education to others is good, but when we seek to convert them to our beliefs by giving them our propaganda in the process, it becomes a poison. It is like giving candy to children to get them under our power.

The Yoga system recognizes that the highest service we can do for the world is our own self-realization. We cannot really improve the world until we have conquered our own inner darkness. In fact, we see throughout history that the greatest harm in the world has usually been done by religious and political fanaticism.

Yoga tells us that the greatest effects are not always the most visible or obvious. A yogi in meditation in the mountains can direct his thought force towards humanity in such a way that he can create more benefit than any number of charitable institutions. Whereas the latter work outwardly at the surface of life, the yogi works inwardly on the source of life. Hence, we need not interpret the solitude and inaction of the yogi as a lack of compassion. It is the same thing as with a king. The king on his throne can direct the affairs of a kingdom without leaving his palace. So too, the yogi in meditation can channel peace to the world without leaving his meditation room. Hence, many yogis prefer to live in areas free of distraction or large numbers of people. This affords them a clearer space for directing the energy of consciousness into the world.

Knowledge is itself the highest form of service, as it is only light which has the power to dispel darkness. Our real service in life cannot be measured by the names, forms, numbers and quantities of the outer world. It is not in how much money we give to charity or how many schools or hospitals we build but how much of the energy of the Divine we bring into life through our own consciousness.

Yogis merge into the Self of all beings, into the Divine being himself. As such, they gain the power to influence all beings from within. Once this is acquired, they need no longer keep a particular body to do benefit to the world. Such yogis become an eternal presence and learn to work through the whole of life. The great teachers are always with us, in nature, in our hearts.

THE YOGA OF TECHNIQUE
Kriya Yoga

The third of the these paths is the Yoga of Technique or inner action (Kriya Yoga). Kriya means action in Sanskrit, particularly the internal actions done on the body and mind to aid the process of meditation. This term is found in the Yoga Sutras as its definition of the practice of Yoga. It is said to consist of three parts: tapas, the energization of the will, svadhyaya, self-study, and Ishwara-pranidhana, surrender to God or the Self-existent power. This definition of the practice of Yoga includes all three methods of jnana (self-study), bhakti (surrender to God) and technique (energization of the will).

All Yoga involves some sort of practice, system or discipline. In the Yogas of Knowledge and Devotion, however, the techniques are subordinated to a more primary self-observation or self-surrender. In general, technique is always secondary in Yoga, because Yoga aims at the realization of the Self or Spirit which is beyond form and action. Technique applies only to the realm of nature or matter. Pure spirit or pure consciousness is beyond all techniques. Technique can help balance our outer nature to bring us to the point of inner awakening, but technique cannot work by itself. It can set the stage, but it is not the main action. Without awareness or devotion technique soon becomes mechanical and can thereby become only another bondage to the mind. Hence, the pursuit of technique as an end in itself is contrary to the path of Yoga.

Yoga uses technique (nature) to go beyond technique (nature). It harmonizes the outer aspects of our nature through various methods to allow us to move beyond them to our inner Being. Yet much of what we consider inner, which may in fact be internal to our ordinary consciousness and activity, like the astral and causal planes, is also external from the standpoint of pure awareness. For this reason techniques can open many internal domains for our minds and help us develop many subtle powers and faculties. This may be useful for our inner growth but can become an obstacle if we get attached to these subtle powers or experiences.

Yoga emphasizes the natural as opposed to the artificial. Hence, its techniques are various ways of awakening ourselves to our nature and attuning ourselves to our actual state. Hence, yoga techniques attempt to return our body, mind, breath and senses to their natural state by exercises aimed at releasing the tension and stress which disrupts them.

The Yogas of Devotion and Knowledge often do better with the support of various techniques. This is particularly true in the modern world wherein we seldom have the physical presence of great teachers or the atmosphere of ashrams to give a good environment for our meditation. To proceed without techniques may be to neglect what is usually a helpful aid, even though it may be overemphasized or abused by the immature.

It is hard for us to go directly to the Divine, but we can always do some action on body or mind to improve or advance our condition. We may not be able to silence the mind or surrender to God, but we can always do a chant, asana or pranayama. We may not be able to do pure or formless meditation but we can meditate upon a form or idea.

The Yogas of Technique are the most diverse in nature, as technique always tends towards differentiation. They are the most complex, though not all are difficult. As many involve the arousing or manipulation of subtle psychic forces, they can be the most dangerous. By this same reason they require more direct guidance, often a living teacher who has mastered the particular technique.

Hatha Yoga

The most basic of the technical Yogas is Hatha Yoga, what we could call the Yoga of the physical body. Its main tools are postures (asanas) and breath (pranayama). It aims at physical health, vitality and longevity, not necessarily spiritual realization. It is the most popular form of Yoga known in the West. Indeed, many of us think that Yoga is nothing but a series of strange physical postures. We should note carefully that no classical text describes Yoga in terms of posture or asana. The main classical text on Yoga, the *Yoga Sutras,* only discusses postures in three out of its two hundred verses.

Nevertheless, the science of asanas is important. For many it is the first step on the path of Yoga, the easiest point of entry. Seeing the yogic wisdom in treating the physical body often helps us to pursue it into the realms of the mind. The principles of right action and conscious movement we learn in Hatha Yoga can be applied on the deeper levels of our being with similar harmonizing effects. The body is not only the beginning of the path of Yoga, it is often the end. Only what we have brought into our physical existence is fully understood and realized. Hence, it is not good to neglect the physical body in our inner searching.

In terms of many Yoga systems, complex asanas are not usually required. For the Yoga of Knowledge or Devotion only the ability to sustain a comfortable sitting pose is necessary. This can be done by sitting comfortably in a chair. It does not require the lotus pose, though it can be helpful, as can siddhasana.

Nor is the proper method of Hatha Yoga to force or strain ourselves into some ideal posture. Its true method is to aid us in gradually relaxing and letting go of all stress and tension in the physical body. It is not a sport that aims at achievement but a form of meditation aiming at peace. Its goal is not to make us more physically conscious but to make us less identified with the physical body by no longer straining at physical movement.

Prana Yoga

Prana Yoga refers to systems that use primarily the breath as a means of controlling the mind. They are the subtler side of Hatha Yoga. The deeper side of the Prana Yogas comes under Kundalini Yoga, as the Kundalini is nothing but the awakened Prana.

As the practice develops, it is the Prana or life-force itself that does the work, which moves the body into the appropriate asanas and the mind into higher states of consciousness. The greatest Yogis were not those who gained their flexibility through a long period of practice or who gradually molded their bodies into various set asanas. They were those who surrendered to Prana, to the cosmic life-force. The postures of Yoga occur naturally when the Prana is awakened. Through it we find ourselves doing asanas we may not even know and without any personal effort, with a mind perfectly still and at ease. It was only at a later time that asanas were standardized and put in books. Hence, it is more important to awaken our life-energy, our connection with the cosmic life, than it is to seek to change our physical state by molding our bodies into certain postures.

Kundalini Yoga

Kundalini Yoga works with the seed energy of the subtle body, called Kundalini or the Serpent Power. It is said to reside in the root chakra and contain within itself all the power of consciousness. Kundalini has become a relatively familiar term today, and some of us think that spiritual development is only possible through it. It is interesting to note, however, that in many ancient and classical teachings Kundalini was not considered so important and is not always mentioned.

In the Yoga of Knowledge, energy is thought to follow awareness. Therefore, the emphasis is on developing the power of attention. In the Yoga of devotion, energy is thought to follow love. Kundalini may not be recognized apart from the intense power of devotion or attention. In neither of these other two systems of Yoga is any special method for awakening the Kundalini required. It is usually to supplement these two Yogas or in the absence of their full power, that methods to arouse the Kundalini may be used. In this regard Kundalini practices can be an important part of these two paths as well.

It should be noted that Kundalini can be aroused artificially by a willful, forced or egoistic practice. It can also be stimulated by drugs or extreme emotional reactions. If the nature is not purified, the Kundalini may only serve to aggrandize the ego. It tends to magnify our nature, so that if our nature is not yet attuned to the Divine Will, it may magnify our weaknesses. Hence, Kundalini practices do have their possible side-effects and should be done with care. The proper awakening of the Kundalini is through Divine grace. This does not mean that any effort on our part is not useful but that our effort must be to attune ourselves to the grace. Merely to arouse Kundalini is not an end in itself. The goal is to move more deeply into peace. When power is not part of peace, it always becomes destructive. The premature arousing of the Kundalini can burn up the nervous system. It can limit or prevent our spiritual growth for perhaps the rest of our lives.

Kundalini can be used up to the level of the third chakra, or solar plexus, to increase the powers of the ego. According the Vedas and Puranas, even the demons practice Yoga up to this level because it gives them more power. The critical mind of the third chakra often considers itself to be enlightened. It does have the power to see through and control other personalities. It sees the limitations in others. However, it cannot see the Divine presence in others, or its own limitations and usually becomes caught in some process of manipulation. Most false gurus operate on this level.

The arousing of the Kundalini is usually brought about through a coordination of posture, breath and mantra, along with certain visualizations. The Kundalini itself is looked upon as the deity, as the Goddess, the high priestess who leads us into the Divine realms of our higher nature.

Laya Yoga
Nada Yoga
Surat Shabda Yoga

There are many Yogas that teach meditation upon the sound current as the main means of spiritual growth. There is a natural sound that comes forth from the subtle body as it begins to come into function. This sound comes from the Kundalini itself. It is said to originate from the heart chakra of the subtle body, the center of unstruck sound. Usually, the devotee closes his eyes and ears, listens to the internal sounds and meditates on the Divine light from the third eye. This brings about an attunement to the ascending current of knowledge and grace represented by the sound current. Still, it is important to have surrender to the Divine or consciousness of the Self, as these turn this meditation from a form of subtle sensation to an energization of aspiration.

INTEGRAL YOGA
Raja Yoga

All Yogas tend to be integral, as all the yogic paths are related. Though each path moves primarily in one of these directions, usually aspects of the other paths are employed as well. An intensity of devotion may bring about the awakening of knowledge, for example. An awakening of knowledge may lead to the arousing of devotion.

Some Yogas aim very consciously at combining all these different approaches to allow for a complete and full development of the nature. Others, like the Yoga of Knowledge, aim at a more direct and immediate ascent and are not as concerned with a comprehensive approach. They see the comprehensiveness coming naturally from the realization of the Self.

Raja Yoga is the classical system of Yoga of Patanjali in the *Yoga Sutras*. It is a form of integral yoga, as it employs knowledge, devotion and techniques. It is primarily a path of knowledge, however.

Raja Yoga has eight parts or limbs, Ashtanga. These are: Yama (right attitudes), Niyama (right observances), Asana (posture), Pranayama (breath control), Pratyahara (control of the senses), Dharana (attention), Dhyana (meditation) and Samadhi (absorption).

Yama and Niyama each consists of five parts. The Yamas are non-violence, truthfulness, non-stealing, control of sexual energy and non-dependence. The Niyamas are purity, contentment, self-discipline, self-study and surrender to the Divine.

Asana means posture. It is holding a comfortable posture for the purpose of meditation.

Pranayama means literally the expansion of the life-force. It is not simply control of the breath and has nothing to do with the suppression of the breath, which can be dangerous. Our prana is always moving. If we suppress the breath, the prana will move into the nervous system and causes various nervous disorders. Pranayama techniques can be anything that connects us up with the cosmic life-force.

Pratyahara is the control of the senses, which is withdrawal from distraction. It does not mean the suppression of the senses. Nor is it a simple matter of closing one's eyes and ears. It means not being moved by the senses, not having the senses and their impressions rule our minds. Hence, it employs techniques like mantra and visualization to gain control over our reactions to sensory impressions.

Dharana means concentration or attention. It is the ability to constantly direct our mental energy to the object we are examining. It does not mean suppressing other objects from our awareness but to increase our energy of interest and inquiry, our passion to know, so that nothing else can disrupt it.

Dhyana means meditation. It is the capacity to hold our mind on the object of our examination. It is to be like a mirror and reflect the reality of things. Or it is to be like a lake that is still and able to reflect the sky. It is the mind in its natural state of quiescence.

Samadhi means absorption. It is the complete understanding of the nature of the object of our attention in which the observer is one with the observed. It is not some exotic ecstasy, thrilling bliss or magical experience but the joy that comes from peace, wherein the object is merged into the state of seeing.

The first five of these eight limbs are called the outer aspect of Yoga. They are preliminary in nature. The first two, Yama and Niyama, refer to the right attitudes, values and life-style practices necessary to the path of Yoga, its ethical foundation. The next three are the means of control, the outer aspects of our nature, as body, breath and senses.

The last three are called Samyama or integration. They naturally go together. Attention naturally leads to meditation, which results in absorption or the unification of the perceiver and the perceived.

In the process of Yoga various siddhis or occult powers may be attained. They may also arise through the use of drugs and powerful herbs, mantras, or through karma. They are usually considered to be obstacles on the path of Yoga and are usually thought to be avoided. The prime siddhi or attainment of Yoga is the abidance in the state of the seer.

For the practice of Yoga two main qualities are necessary. These are discrimination (viveka) and detachment (vairagya). Discrimination is the ability to discern the difference between truth and falsehood, reality and unreality, the Self and the not-Self, happiness and sorrow, the inner and the outer. Detachment is the ability to release the mind from its mental and emotional biases that serve to color our perception. Detachment leads to renunciation. Renunciation is not giving things up but no longer believing in external realities. It means no longer investing name and form with any ultimate reality but seeing the sacred presence as the real being and value of things.

The goal of Yoga is to return to the inner Self or the Divine, the Purusha. To do this we must seperate from the outer process of the world, Prakriti. We must cease to identify ourselves with any external state or quality. Eventually, we must detach our sense of identity from the thoughts of the mind, from our very self-image itself. We must return to the state of the Seer, to the state of pure seeing in which all is one and one is all. This is not to abandon the world but to no longer see it as possessing any seperate reality, to see it as a play of consciousness rather than an external thing.

EXPERIENCE IN YOGA

Yoga can provide us with many subtle and dramatic experiences. We may hear special sounds or see special colors. We may do astral travel or visit other worlds. We may contact beings of these other worlds, who may speak through us. We may connect up with souls of the past or the future. Yet the goal of Yoga is not to gain any particular experience. Rather, it is freedom from experience that is the goal of Yoga. Yoga aims at deconditioning the mind, and each experience has the power to condition the mind should we cling to it or invest it with some personal energy. Subtle experiences can bind the mind even more so than normal sensory experiences, as their reality is harder to judge.

Hence, when experiences arise in Yoga, one should observe them objectively but hold to the awareness or state of grace. Yoga is to merge us into the Divine or the inner Self, not merely to open us up to other forms of experience. Many great Yogis may have no experiences at all but only a greater awareness or sense of love. For Yoga it is not the form or appearance that matters but the essence. We need not feel bad if we do not gain great experiences on the path of Yoga.

THE ASTRAL PLANE

Most subtle experiences gained in Yoga come through the astral plane, the realm of imagination. On the astral plane, whatever we imagine about ourselves we can experience as true. Hence, the astral plane is the realm of illusion. While the Divine can be reached through the higher astral plane, we can also find the Divine in the waking state without ever opening up to the astral. We can open up to the causal plane (formless realm) directly, so as to avoid the dangers of the astral.

YOGA, SHAMANISM AND CHANNELING

Yoga is one means of exploring the occult realms of nature. This, however, is not the main focus of Yoga, which is to go beyond nature, but a sidelight. There are other means of exploring these subtle realms, as in magic, occultism and shamanism. These things can be part of a subtler form of science wherein we discover the hidden forces behind the world. There is nothing wrong with exploring them, but they are still only phenomenal.

The higher forms of Shamanism move in the direction of Yoga. They aim at a greater development of awareness and self-knowledge, towards the liberation of the Spirit from all bondage to the external. The lower forms of Shamanism, however, may get us caught in the illusions of the astral plane. This is particularly true if they employ drugs, if they aim at the accumulation of personal power rather than the surrender to the Divine, if they awaken animal forces within us, if they are centered on the solar plexus and below rather than the heart. In this regard they are like the left-handed yogic paths which can become forms of black magic.

Channeling often involves having another being or entity speak through us. In Yoga the emphasis is on self-knowledge and the development of our own awareness. Yoga says that we should never give our awareness over to another person or entity, internally or externally. We should never surrender the integrity of our own individual awareness because that is the Divine presence within us. If our channeling is based on a loss of consciousness, such channeling is a detriment to our own inner growth, though it may provide information that others find useful. We read little about channeling in Yogic literature, except channeling the flow of Divine grace.

It is the Divine or our own inner Self that we should channel and such higher qualities as love and compassion, but to do that is an act of consciousness, not the letting of another being work through us. We should all be channels for the Gods or the cosmic powers, to lead us back to our own divinity. Yoga tells us that we can communicate directly to the Divine. The Divine is our inner Self. We need no intermediary. Even the guru is not an intermediary that inhibits us from our own direct contact with the Divine. His role is as a facilitater or catalyst who helps us in this process of self-knowing.

While it is necessary as a culture that we once more link up to the astral plane and come to understand the occult forces in nature, this is only a beginning to a greater understanding of the spiritual nature of life. It is only connecting to the subtle plane nearest our own. It is not going to the truth. We can also go directly to the source of all creation. It dwells in our own hearts as the light behind the mind. The Yogic path does not rest content with lesser goals.

HIGH TECH YOGAS

A new approach to Yoga has been arising today in the modern and technological world, what is called "high tech" Yoga. High tech Yogas try to use the means of technology as part of the practice of Yoga. They may involve watching special videos, listening to subliminal tapes, using equipment or machines to stimulate the brain and senses or alter the brain waves, etc.

Their form is generally passive. We watch or listen to something, or let someone or some machine work on our energy, and it is supposed to have an elevating affect upon us or even bring us to enlightenment. While such things may be helpful in working with the outer aspects of our nature, they have their limitations in the realm of spiritual practices. Even in healing the body, inorganic energies, which is what machines produce, can have a deranging affect upon the life-force, or prana. True Yoga practice is never passive. Passivity creates fragmentation and disintegration. Integration is only possible through cultivating our own direct experience and creative process in life, not in what is gained second hand.

Subliminal messages can be a form of hypnosis and a violation of our consciousness. They encourage a state of unconsciousness and wishful thinking. We are already too hypnotized, too dominated by suggestions and external conditioning influences, particularly those of the mass media. We cannot become a great artist merely by listening to a tape that says "you are a great artist." We have to have the inspiration and do the work if we would get the results. Subliminal messages can be a subtle form of violence. They may cover over what we are with an artificial idea from the outside, not connect us with the truth within us, which can only come through consciousness.

We must remember that the medium is always the message. The message may be God or truth, but if the medium is passively watching a video, using subliminal suggestions or channeling, what we are actually encouraging is the unconsciousness of the medium, the dependence on external stimulation. Yoga is not a form of entertainment or self-hypnosis. While high tech Yogas may be interesting or even fun, we should be aware of the limitation of reliance on external stimulation. They may give us a reflection of certain Yogic states but they may not be the means to gain them.

True Yoga practice is not a matter of a special technology, of having the best tapes, books or latest equipment. Its essence is in simplicity and in allying ourselves with the forces of nature. It is something we must do for ourselves, by disciplining our own body, mind and senses according to a higher aspiration. No one can practice Yoga for us or give us Yoga from the outside, anymore than anyone can breathe for us. Yoga, on the contrary, is freeing ourselves from any dependence on external programming.

12
THE SOURCE TEACHINGS
THE VEDAS, PURANAS AND TANTRAS

The One Truth the sages call by many names.
— Rig Veda I. 164.

There are many different forms of spiritual and religious teachings in the world devised to lead us to the truth. The Hindu and Vedic teaching contains all possible varieties of these.

Each religion has its source teaching. These are usually called scriptures. The Judeao-Christian teaching has the *Bible*, Islam, the *Koran*, Buddhism has the Buddha's Sutras, Taoism has the *Tao Teh Ching*, and Zoroastrianism, the *Zend Avesta*. The *Bible* and *Koran* consist of ancient history, stories and symbolic teachings. The Buddhist Sutras are mainly the lectures and discourses of the Buddha and possess a philosophical nature. They are also a more diverse body than the scriptures of these other religions. The *Tao Teh Ching* is the sayings of Lao Tse. The *Zend Avesta* consists of the prayers of Zarathustra.

Hinduism does not contain any central source teaching like these. There is no simple bible all must study or follow every day. The ancient Vedas have a similar position theoretically as scriptures, we might say, but they are seldom read or understood today, and are a far more diverse set of teachings from a number of different sources and teachers. For source teachings today each sect of Hinduism has its own scriptures. Most of these derive from various Puranas, *Agama*s and Tantras, not from the older Veda, though they are still based upon the Vedas and quote from them for their authority.

Let us imagine that we make today a great scripture combining the teachings of the great sages, prophets and avatars of the world. We would have sections in it on all the world's great religions, the names of many sages, many different names for the Divine and many different approaches to it. We would have Christian, Judaic, Islamic, Hindu, Buddhist and Taoist teachings. If we were more eclectic or broad minded we would include Shinto, Zoroastrian, Native American, African, Polynesian and perhaps even teachings of religions which have passed away like those of ancient Greece, Egypt and Babylonia.

Now, if someone at some point in the future found such a book, not knowing its origin or scope, perhaps not having a clear idea as to what the words mean, they could make many wrong conclusions. They might consider such a great universal scripture is teaching polytheism as the names of God are so many. They could assume it was a product of a limited local culture and reduce these names of the Divine to different tribal Gods. In this way Allah could be considered the God of one tribe, Buddha that of another, Christ that of a third and so on.

This is what has been done to the Vedas (and many other ancient teachings) by modern scholarship. Its terms for the Divine, which all have a general as well as specific meaning, become the names of local or limited Gods. A universalist approach is reduced to a multiplistic one. The ancient names for different Gods are in their truest sense only different names for God.

Some of us may say it is hard to believe the ancients had such a broad approach to the Divine as to have conceived of a single Divine with many attributes. After all their cultures were much more limited than ours and not always in very good communication with each other. Their understanding and control of the material world appears quite limited as well. Why should we think they had a better grasp of the infinite and the eternal?

On the other hand, their cultures did last much longer than ours, some enduring for thousands of years relatively unchanged like that of ancient Egypt. Their focus was much more on the realm of religion than ours. Our modern archaeologists find their ruins filled with fetishes and objects of worship possessing a ritualistic rather than a practical value. Moreover, knowledge or skill in the material world does not necessarily include that of the spiritual realm, so a lack of it may not exclude it either. Hence, the ancients could very well have had quite a diversity of religious or spiritual approaches, even in a small area. Look at the philosophical diversity we find in great ages of humanity like ancient Greece, though the land itself was rather small. So too, we cannot judge the breadth of ideas by the material limitations of a culture.

Probably the most universal and comprehensive of such ancient teachings is the *Rig Veda,* the oldest teaching of India. It is not surprising that it has been reduced to such a polytheistic interpretation, though it states in many places the unity of truth and the identity of one God with all the Gods.

The basis of all scriptures is a rendering into human language of the Word of God. It is not our culture alone which has a book it claims to be the word of God. All cultures have them. Some have many such books. The word of God is called mantra in Sanskrit. By the spiritual origin and power of the Sanskrit language many mantric or scriptural texts thus exist within it. The most primary is the source book of the mantra, the *Rig Veda*.

THE BOOK OF MANTRA
THE VEDAS

The Vedas are the ancient scriptures or revelation (Shruti) of the Hindu teachings. They manifest the Divine Word in human speech. They reflect into human language the language of the Gods, the Divine powers which have created us and which rule over us.

There are four Vedas, each consisting of four parts. The primary portion is the mantra or hymn section (samhita). To this are appended ritualistic teachings (brahmana) and theological sections (aranyaka). Finally, philosophical sections (upanishads) are included.

The hymn sections are the oldest. The others were added at a later date, and each explains some aspect of the hymns or follows one line of interpreting them. The Vedas were compiled around the time of Krishna (c. 1500 B.C.), and even at that time were hardly understood. Hence, they are very ancient and only in recent times has their spiritual import, like that of the other mystery teachings of the ancient world, begun to be rediscovered or appreciated. Like the Egyptian teachings, they are veiled, symbolic and subtle and require a special vision to understand and use properly.

The great compiler of the Vedas and Puranas was Vyasa Krishna Dwaipayana. He was said to be the twenty-eighth of the Vyasas or compilers of Vedic knowledge. He was somewhat older than the Avatar Krishna, and his work continued after the death of Krishna. Perhaps he is symbolic of a whole Vedic school which flourished at that time, as many such Vedic schools were once prominent all over India and in some places beyond.

THE RIG VEDA
THE SOURCE BOOK OF MANTRA

The *Rig Veda* is the oldest of the Vedas. All the other Vedas are based upon it and consist to a large degree of various hymns from it. It consists of a thousand such hymns of different seers, each hymn averaging around ten verses. The *Rig Veda* is the oldest book in Sanskrit or any Indo-European language. Its date is debatable. Many great Yogis and scholars, who have understood the astronomical references in the hymns, date the *Rig Veda* as before 4000 B.C., perhaps as early as 12,000 B.C.. Modern western scholars tend to date it around 1500 B.C., though recent archeological finds in India now appear to require a much earlier date. While the term Vedic is often given to any layer of the Vedic teachings including the *Bhagavad Gita,* technically it applies primarily to the *Rig Veda.*

The *Rig Veda* is the book of Mantra. It contains the oldest form of all the Sanskrit mantras. It is built around a science of sound which comprehends the meaning and power of each letter. Most aspects of Vedic science, like the practice of Yoga, meditation, mantra and Ayurveda can be found in the *Rig Veda* and still use many terms that come from it. While originally several different versions or rescensions of the *Rig Veda* were said to exist, only one remains. Its form has been structured in several different ways to guarantee its authenticity and proper preservation through time.

The *Rig Veda* consists of the hymns to various aspects of the Divine as seen by various seers, called the rishis. There are seven primary seers, identified, not only in India but also in Persia and China, with the seven stars of the Big Dipper. Their names are Atri, Kanwa, Vasishta, Vishwamitra, Jamadagni, Gotama and Bharadvaja, but they appear even in the hymns of these sages and may refer to an earlier group. They relate to the guiding lights of the seven chakras.

The main family of the seers was called the Angirasas (a term related to the Greek Angelos and our English word angel). The seven seers are all Angirasas and their families or lineages are a diversification of this one original line. The foremost of the Angirasas was Brihaspati, identified with the planet Jupiter. Other important seer families were the Bhrigus (associated with Venus) and the Ribhus. Some Vedic Gods may have also been families of the seers, including the Maruts, the Adityas and the Ashwins.

Each of the seven seer families still has many descendants in India and elsewhere. They were said to be the progenitors of the human race. The head of each of the seer families was like a Tulku and took many births or passed on his teaching to many successors who bore his name. Hence, Vedic and Puranic literature is filled with many Vasishtas, Vishwamitras, etc.

The *Rig Veda* is composed of ten books (called mandalas in Sanskrit). Seven of the books each relate primarily to one great seer and the family he belongs to; the second book belongs to Gritsamada and his family, the Bhrigus; the third relates to Vishwamitra and his family; the fourth to Vamadeva and the Gotama family; the fifth to Atri and his family; the sixth to Bharadvaja and his family; the seventh to Vasishta and his family; and the eighth to the Kanwas. The first book is a collection of hymns from seers of different families, mainly earlier ones. The tenth book is a collection of various earlier and later hymns. The ninth book is the collection of Soma hymns, mainly from the Bhrigus and Angirasas. It is largely outside of and earlier than the family books. Hence, the Soma book is the oldest of them all.

Each hymn is given to a certain deity (devata). The main deities are Indra, Agni, Soma and Surya. The Vedic Gods have many different levels of meaning. They represent an intuitive symbology which transcends the limited constructs of the intellectual mind.

Indra is the God of Prana or the awakened life-force. He represents the perceiver or the consciousness of the seer. He is the young warrior wielding the thunderbolt or vajra, which destroys the demons or powers of falsehood. Agni is the God of consciousness, awareness and mindfulness. His symbol is the sacred fire. The outer offerings to him symbolize our inward giving to the higher awareness within us. Soma is the mystic plant that yields the nectar of immortality. He is also the Moon and the lord of the waters. He symbolizes bliss, Ananda. Surya is the Sun which is the visible face and presence of the Deity. He symbolizes the enlightened mind and creative intelligence. He is the Divine creator and transformer.

Other important deities are Varuna, the lord of the cosmic ocean and the Divine judge; Mitra, the Divine friend and lord of compassion; and Savitar, the Sun God of creative intelligence. Goddesses are Usha, the Goddess of the Dawn or spiritual aspiration; Saraswati, the Goddess of the Divine Word, of wisdom and inspiration; Aditi, the Goddess of Infinite Oneness and Wholeness; and Apas, the Cosmic Waters. Moreover, each of the Gods has his consort, like Indra and Indrani, Varuna and Varunani. Collective deities exist like the Adityas, the solar deities, the Maruts or Rudras, Gods of the storm, the Ribhus or Divine craftsmen and the Vishvedevas, literally the universal Gods who symbolize the unity of all the Gods.

The trinity of later Hinduism, Brahma the creator, Vishnu the maintainer and Shiva the destroyer is present in the *Rig Veda* but behind the scenes. Brahma is Brihaspati, also called Brahmanaspati, the priest of the Gods. Vishnu is an important form of the Sun God, and later all forms of the Sun God were merged into him. Shiva is present as Rudra, the seldom invoked but very much respected and feared father of all the Gods.

Each God or Goddess represents certain Divine qualities. They are present as the guiding forces, both in nature and in the human psyche. Hence, they are largely a personification of ideas, of the truth perceptions, the great archetypes of the Divine Mind. For example, the God Mitra, whose name literally means friend, stands for friendship and its importance in life as a divine or spiritual quality.

Each God or Goddess can be any or all the Gods. The concepts of monotheism, polytheism, pantheism and monism are all woven together in the Vedic vision of totality. The Divine is seen as both One and Many without contraction. The Divine is all the universe and all the cosmic powers which rule it, but it also transcends the world. Such a wholistic view of the world was quite confusing to the scholars who first translated the Vedas, but perhaps today we can appreciate it better in light of our larger view of the world and the psyche.

THE SAMA VEDA
THE MYSTIC SONG

The *Sama Veda* is the Yoga of Song. It consists of various hymns of the *Rig Veda* put to a different and more musical chant. Hence, the text of the *Sama Veda* is a reduced version of the *Rig Veda*. Its secret is in its musical annotation and rendering.

The *Sama Veda* represents the ecstasy of spiritual knowledge and the power of devotion. The *Rig Veda* is the word, the *Sama Veda* is the song or the meaning. The *Rig Veda* is the knowledge, the *Sama Veda* its realization. Hence, the two always go together like husband and wife. The *Rig Veda* is the wife and the *Sama Veda* is the husband.

THE YAJUR VEDA
THE MYSTIC RITUAL

The *Yajur Veda* seen by the outer vision is the Veda of ritual. On an inner level, it sets forth a yogic practice for purifying the mind and awakening the inner consciousness. Several versions of the *Yajur Veda* exist, which differ in a number of respects. It was the main Veda used by the priests in ancient India and has much in common with the *Egyptian Book of the Dead*.

Its deities are the same as the *Rig Veda*. The purpose of the ritual is to put together and recreate within ourselves the Cosmic Man or Indra. The ritual is to recreate the universe within our own psyche and thereby unite the individual with the universal. Its series of sacrifices culminates in the Atmayajna or the self-sacrifice wherein the ego is offered up to the Divine. While the lesser sacrifices win the lesser worlds, the Self-sacrifice wins all the worlds and gains the greatest gift of immortality.

THE ATHARVA VEDA

The *Atharva Veda* is the last of the Vedas. It has not always been accepted as a Veda, which are often spoken of as three. It still contains many hymns from the *Rig Veda* but also has some more popular magic spells which are outside of the strictly ritual-knowledge orientation of the other Vedas. Like the *Rig Veda,* it is a collection of hymns but of a more diverse character, most very exalted like the *Rig Veda,* but reflecting a more common language. As such, it gives us a better idea of the life of common people in Vedic times.

The deities of the *Atharva Veda* are also the same as the *Rig Veda,* although Rudra-Shiva assumes a more visible role. The language is a little simpler and less variable in its forms.

Atharvan is also an important figure in the Zoroastrian religion. Atar is the Persian name for fire, and the Atharvan is the fire priest.

THE BOOK OF KNOWLEDGE
UPANISHADS

Upanishad means the inner or mystic teaching. The Upanishads more clearly set forth the prime Vedic doctrines, like Self-realization, Yoga and meditation, karma and reincarnation, which were hidden or kept veiled under the symbols of the older mystery religion. The older Upanishads are usually affixed to a particularly Veda, through a Brahmana or Aranyaka (see below). The more recent ones are not. The Upanishads became prevalent some centuries before the time of Krishna and Buddha. The classical Upanishadic age was in the reign of the Kuru kings of north India, before the time of Krishna (c. 1500 B.C.).

Perhaps the most proment figure in the Upanishads is the sage Yajnavalkya. Most of the great teachings of later Hindu and Buddhist philosophy derive from him. He taught the great doctrine of neti-neti, the view that truth can be found only through the negation of all thoughts about it. He looks back some generations to Tura Kavasheya, the main priest of Janamejaya, the third of the Kuru kings (not to be confused with the later Janamejaya who followed a few generations after Krishna). Other important Upanishadic sages are: Uddalaka Aruni, Shwetaketu, Shandilya, Aitareya, Pippalada, and Sanat Kumara. Many earlier Vedic teachers like Manu, Brihaspati, Ayasya and Narada are also found in the Upanishads. Upanishads often quote verses from the *Rig Veda* to support their declarations of spiritual knowledge.

In the Upanishads the spiritual meanings of the Vedic texts are brought out and emphasized in their own right. More specifically, the Upanishads are a development from the *Sama Veda* and continue to emphasize the ecstasy and the realization of the revealed knowledge of the Vedas. Some Upanishadic teachings can be found in the *Atharva Veda* as well. Most Upanishadic ideas are found in the *Rig Veda,* though it follows a different type of expression.

The classical Upanishads are the *Brihadaranyaka, Chandogya, Isha, Aitareya, Taittiriya, Katha, Prashna, Kena, Mundaka, Mandukya,* and

Shwetasavatara. These were given commentaries by great philosopher
Shankara many centuries later. Probably all of these Upanishads and some
others as well are pre-Buddhist in nature. Upanishads continued to be
written into fairly recent times and now several hundred exist.

The *Bhagavad Gita* of Sri Krishna is considered by many to be an
Upanishad, as it is a summary of their teachings. The Upanishads are said
to be the cows, with Krishna their milker and the *Gita* the milk.

The basic teachings of the Upanishads are summed up in six great
sayings (Mahavakyas). These are:

1) I am Brahman (Aham Brahmasmi). This states the identity of the
inmost consciousness of the individual with that of the supreme
Divine. The ultimate truth of Vedic knowledge is not that some great
saviour is God or the Lord, or that such and such a God or name and
form of God is the supreme. It is not the worship of a person, book,
image or idea. It is not even the worship of God. The Upanishads say
that whatever we worship as truth, apart from ourselves, destroys us.
They teach that our own Self is the true Divinity, that it is the presence
of the absolute within our heart and all the universe.

2) The Self is Brahman (Ayam Atma Brahma). This also states the
identity of the soul with the Absolute but in a more objective and less
direct manner. Not only is our Self the Divine. It is the same Self in
all beings that is the same Absolute truth.

3) That thou art (Tat tvam asi). Whatever we see or think about, we
are that. Not only is the I That, the You is also That. We are that
ultimate I and Thou in all. The consciousness in the other is also the
Divine.

4) Intelligence is Brahman (Prajnanam Brahma). Our discernment
of truth is the truth itself. It indicates that the Divine intelligence is
present within us and has the power to return us to the Divine. Our
inmost intelligence is that supreme intelligence through which we
can merge into the Absolute.

5) All the Universe is Brahman (Sarvam Khalvidam Brahma). The
entire universe is the Divine, which includes our self. The Divine is
not only the consciousness principle in you and I, it is also the being
principle in all things. It is the ultimate object as well as the inmost
subject in all beings. It is one in all and all in one.

6) He am I (So'ham). This shows the identity of the self with the
Divine Lord inherent within the natural movement of our breath. So
is the natural sound of inhalation, ham of exhalation.

These great sayings are much like the I am that I am of the *Bible* but more clearly articulated. They are statements of the identity of the individual consciousness with the Absolute or Divine reality. They all derive from and merge into Om, the Divine Word "I am all."

THE BOOK OF RITUAL
THE BRAHMANAS

The *Brahmanas* are specific ritualistic texts, and were often used by the great priests in the courts of the Aryans kings. They are much like the *Yajur Veda* and its ritualistic approach but are not as old, nor do they have such an esoteric meaning. Yet they are more extensive. They set forth an important system of occult knowledge. They show us how to recreate the ritual action of life itself, to portray the cosmic ritual in a few special actions.

Not all their rituals are of an outward nature. The outer things offered were symbolic of inner processes. The ritual proceeds primarily through speech, breath and mind. The main power of the ritual is the mantra or the chant. The chants attune us to the cosmic vibration and connect us with the transformative force of nature. The ritual brings us into the right action of life. The ritual order, or the order of the sacrifice, is the sacred nature and movement of life. Such rituals and chants prepare us for the spiritual knowledge, make our life and thought a rich field for it to grow. The *Brahmanas* thereby lead us to the Upanishads.

Some Vedic rituals involved animal sacrifices but, on an esoteric level, the animal to be sacrificed is our own lower nature. The *Brahmanas* are opposed to the slaughter of animals except as an occasional sacred rite done with discretion. Contrary to the views of many modern scholars, the Vedic animal sacrifice did not encourage meat-eating or the mistreatment of animals. Rather, it taught the common people, who could not be expected to be vegetarian at that more primitive state of society, the sacred nature of the animal and that it should only be killed as an offering to the Gods. Hence, the animal sacrifice instilled not only a reverence for the sacred but also a respect for animal life, which was seen as belonging to the Gods.

Important *Brahmanas* are the *Aitareya, Shatapatha, Kaushitaki, Taittiriya* and *Chandogya.* They are longer, sometimes much longer, than their respective Upanishads. This is not because they were more important but because their teaching was more complex. However, they repeat a certain set ritual and so are all variations on the same teaching. The rituals were aligned with the seasons and the equinoxes and were the basis for the calendar the culture followed.

THE FOREST TEXTS
THE ARANYAKAS

Between the *Brahmanas* and Upanishads are a few secondary texts. These are called *Aranyakas* or Forest texts to be used by those who left society to reside in the forest to gain spiritual knowledge. They combine ritual passages with philosophical texts and some Upanishads are contained within them or appendiced to them. Important *Aranyakas* are the *Taittiriya, Aitareya* and the *Shankhayana.*

THE BOOK OF MYTH
THE PURANAS

The Puranas are the richest collection of mythology in the world. Most of them attained their final form around 500 A.D., but they were passed on as an oral tradition since the time of Krishna (c. 1500 B.C.).

There are eighteen major Puranas and several minor ones called *Upapuranas.* Each is a long book consisting of various stories of the Gods and Goddesses, hymns, an outline of ancient history, cosmology, rules of life, rituals, instructions on spiritual knowledge. Hence, the Puranas are like encyclopedias of religion and culture and contain material of different levels and degrees of difficulty.

The eighteen Puranas are the *Vishnu, Brahma, Agni, Vayu, Linga, Kurma, Markandeya, Narada, Vamanana, Matsya, Varaha, Skanda, Garuda, Brahmanda, Shri Bhagavata, Bhavishya,* and *Brahmavaivartta.* The *Upapuranas* are *Shiva Purana, Kalki Purana, Kalika Purana,* etc. The most important of these texts are the *Vishnu Purana, Shiva Purana* and *Markandeya Purana.*

The Puranas are perhaps the most important or commonly used scriptural texts of the Hindus. They were guide books for the whole of life and society.

THE BOOK OF LEGEND
ITIHASAS

Along with the Puranas or books of mythology, are the *Itihasas* or books of legend. These are not ordinary legends but refer to the lives of avatars or incarnations of God. Like the Puranas they contain myths and legends but their predomination differs. Two main epics exist, the *Ramayana,* the epic of Rama and Sita, and the *Mahabharata,* by far the longest of all these teachings, which is mainly the story of Krishna. His story is the most dwelt upon subject in the Puranas as well.

Rama is also mentioned in the Persian literature along with the God Vayu (the Wind). Hanuman, the monkey God and Rama's companion was also the God of the Wind. His wife Sita is the Goddess of the Earth, the furrowed ground, from the *Rig Veda.*

THE AGAMAS

The *Agamas* are ancient Shaivite scriptures, of a similar antiquity with the Puranas and Upanishads. They are also extensive, profound and worthy of study and reverence.

TANTRA

Tantra is a well known but highly misunderstood Sanskrit term. Literally, it means a fabric and refers to a whole set of teachings, both Hindu and Buddhist, given in ancient and medieval times, from perhaps a few centuries before Christ until after 1000 A.D. There are many teachings called Tantras with not always a lot in common.

There are three basic levels of teachings in the Vedic dharma. The oldest layer is Vedic, consisting of the Vedas themselves, along with the Upanishads and *Brahmanas.* These were prevalent in ancient times, and were out of vogue some centuries before the time of the Buddha. The second layer is the Puranic, consisting of the Puranas and Epics. These came into prominence at the time of the kings that followed Krishna, as the Vedic teaching declined, but are considered an extension and development of the Vedas. They continued in the forefront until about 500 A.D., though they are still commonly used. The third is the Tantra. It is a development and extension of the Puranas and legends, and is not as clearly differentiated from them, as they are from the Vedas. An important Tantra is the *Mahanirvana.*

Tantra has become more well known in the West than the other Vedic teachings mainly for the sexual Tantras, those giving various sexual practices for attaining ecstasy, union with God or awakening the Kundalini. These, in fact, are quite rare among the Tantras and are not at all indicative of them as a whole.

Tantra has also been associated with the worship of the Goddess. It is true that there are many Tantric teachings to the Goddess. Yet there are many Tantras to the Gods, like Shiva and Vishnu; hence, Tantra, as such, cannot be equated with Goddess worship. On the whole, the Tantras do not give the Goddess any more prominent a place than other levels of the Vedic and Hindu teachings, as the Goddess is important in all levels of the teaching.

Tantra has also been associated with energy teachings and practices. These include mantra, yantra, visualization, rituals and pujas. While such practices are often more specifically Tantric, they can be found in all layers of the Vedic and Puranic teachings. Tantra has been specifically linked to the development of Kundalini. Kundalini does play a more prominent place in the Tantras than in the Vedas and Puranas. In these earlier teachings the emphasis is more on knowledge (jnana) or devotion (bhakti), and less on techniques. But there are also Tantras which emphasize knowledge or devotion, while technical practices are sometimes given in the Vedas and Puranas (though these were more part of an oral tradition as they had to be adopted for each individual).

YANTRA

Yantra is the use of various energy patterns, or geometrical designs. The Yantra is the energy form of the mantra. It is the subtle form of the deity. Yantras are used not only for visualization and meditation, but also used for good luck, like talismans. They help us redirect our psychic energy in a creative and transformative manner. Many astrologers prescribe them, and they are as useful, though less expensive than gems, for warding off negative planetary influences.

Most important is the Shri Yantra, the main yantra to the Goddess. Other important yantras are Ganesh Yantra for giving good fortune and warding off obstacles and Mahamrityunjaya Yantra for warding off death and difficulties. Special Yantras exist for each of the planets.

Mandalas are extended yantras. Around various yantras additional forms, usually of Gods and Goddesses, are added. Mandalas are also mainly for meditation and are prominent in the Buddhist tradition.

SUMMARY OF THE SOURCE TEACHINGS

These and other source teachings can be divided into several categories: 1) The Book of Mantra or the Divine Word, 2) The Book of Ritual, 3) The Book of Mythology, 4) The Book of Legend, and 5) The Book of Knowledge or the Inner teaching.

In the Vedic Dharma, the Vedic hymns, particularly those of the *Rig Veda,* are the Mantra which is the basic scripture from which the others evolve, the poetry from which they grow. The Ritual is represented by the *Brahmanas* and the *Yajur Veda.* Mythology is represented by the Puranas. Legend is represented by the *Itihasas.* The Book of Knowledge is represented by the Upanishads. The Tantras are composite in nature but could be considered as the Book of Techniques or practices.

In the universal religion the forms of these may vary according to the differences of time, place and culture, but all source teachings must come in one or another of these categories, or contain them on different levels of interpretation. In this regard any real mantra is a Vedic hymn, any true myth a Purana, any realization of truth an Upanishad. All the other spiritual or religious teachings of the world can be placed in one of these categories. The existent texts are but examples of these different modes of teaching and methods of communication to the different levels of our mind and aspects of our being. It is important, therefore, that we continue all these lines of teaching, but we must creatively adapt their forms. We need not merely worship old texts. We must continue their energy with renewed intensity.

SACRED HISTORY AND COSMOLOGY

Particularly in the Puranas and *Itihasas*, we find presented the Vedic view of human history and of the order of the universe. We do find some of what we might consider from our rationalistic perspective to represent human history or a description of the physical world. However, we find many mythic elements which appear quite imaginary. For example, the Earth is said to consist of seven continents divided by seven seas of different substances like water, milk, honey, etc.

Such views, however, were never meant to portray the actual state of things in time and space. They include not just the visible world in their scope but also the invisible worlds.

Sacred history is not concerned with the actual dates of various events. It is concerned with showing how we fell from the eternal into time and how we can return from time to the eternal. It shows where the eternal intersects time. It may also consider how time in our world is connected with time in the other more subtle worlds. Whereas our secular history is linear, sacred history has a qualitative dimension that cuts through chronological time at only one level. The wars between the Gods and demons, the positive and negative forces of the cosmos, appear in this as important as or as behind the wars on Earth.

Sacred cosmology, similarly, is not concerned with the actual location of places on Earth. It shows how the sacred is reflected into our environment. It does not judge things by their actual size but the degree to which the sacred comes through them. This may be determined by cultural or psychic as well as physical factors. A sacred mountain may not actually be the highest mountain, but its sacred dimension makes it larger in the perspective of sacred cosmology. The individual who transcribed such accounts was not a victim of false imagination or wrong measurement but was judging things by a different standard. Sacred space interpenetrates secular space at various points. In these points ordinary dimensions disappear and the miraculous or magical can be found.

For example, in the Vedic tradition, the sacred mountain at the center of the world called Kailas or Meru, is said to be at the north pole and the source of the four rivers which support the world. Most cultures have their mythic world mountain. Kailas is identified with a mountain in Tibet, north of the Himalayan range. Such an identification is symbolic or mythical. Actually, any mountain can be the sacred mountain. Mount Meru in Tibet may not be at the actual north pole, nor is it the highest mountain in the world. But it may still be at the spiritual north pole of the world. Its sacred dimension may give it a quality that makes it the highest and most central mountain in the world. It may be the home of many Divine teachers, perhaps the Lord of the World on the subtle planes. In all these things it is the inner meaning we must look to and not just simply look down upon other cultures because they were not speaking in our language.

Such sacred languages have their place in life. They are not to be interpreted literally, though they may have some relevance to the outer scheme of things. To insist they are literally true or to deny them because they are not is a failure of intelligence, the application of a wrong standard. To understand life we must return to the sacred vision such as we find in the Vedas that makes the inner dimension of life rule over the outer, but which gives each its appropriate place.

The way to enter into sacred time is through participation in the ritual. The ritual occurs according to the sacred calendar. It celebrates the life of the deity or the avatar. Through it we leave our petty personal time wherein we are caught in the affairs of the outer world and participate inwardly in the life of the universe. The way to enter into sacred space is to enter into a temple or other sacred place. This is to leave the world of territory and possession and enter the domain of the infinite.

Hence, scriptures always seek to incarnate themselves in temples and religious festivals. These are the scripture or source teaching in manifestation in the outer world. In the world of the mind they manifest through study, chanting and meditation. This living application is their real power and existence which we should maintain and which we must maintain to keep our lives in harmony with the Divine.

APPENDICES

SELECTIONS FROM
VEDIC TEACHINGS

While adequate modern translation of many Hindu and Vedic teachings exist, for the ancient texts little is yet available that shows them in their true proportions. The modern mind has yet to penetrate the veil protecting the ancient mysteries. Hence, I have given some glimpses of these source teachings here. The great teachings of yoga were contained in the Vedic teachings from the beginning. In the course of time the language of the teachings changed, but the basic truth has continued like an undying flame.

RIG VEDA
Mandala I, Sukta 1
Seer — Madhucchandas, Deity — Agni

This hymn, which is used to open the collection of the hymns of the *Rig Veda,* is a typical chant to the fire of awareness and mindfulness (Agni) which ever has been the foundation of meditation and the path of yoga.

1. I give energy to the Fire of Consciousness that is placed before all things, the Divinity of the sacrifice who acts in the season of truth, the invoker best to establish the ecstasy.

2. The Fire adored by the ancient seers is adored again by the new. Into our presence he brings the Gods.

3. Through the Flame of Awareness one attains to a reality which increases in nourishment every day, a glory full of heroic power.

4. Oh Fire, that sacred movement which you pervade from every side, that indeed enters into the Divine.

5. The Fire, the invoker, the seer-will, the truth, the most revelatory knowledge, Divine he comes with all that is Divine.

6. Oh Fire, whatever auspicious you create for the mortal who harmonizes himself to you, that is your Truth, oh perceiving ray.

7. To you, oh Fire, day by day, by night and by dawn, bearing our surrender we come,

8. The King of the sacred movement, the guardian of truth, increasing in his self-nature every day.

9. So, as a father to his son, be of easy access to us, hold closely to us for our well-being.

SHUKLA YAJUR VEDA
CHAPTER 32

This is one of the more obviously mystical of the forty chapters of the white *Yajur Veda*. The others have a similar meaning but more veiled by the symbolism of the ritual.

1. That alone is the Fire, That is the Sun, That is the Wind and That alone the Moon. That is the luminous seed, That the Supreme Reality, That is the cosmic Waters and the Lord of Creation.

2. All vibrations took birth from the lightning Spirit. Nothing can encompass him above, below or in the middle.

3. He has no image, whose name is great glory.

4. He is the God who exists in all directions. The ancient One, he takes birth within the child. He is what has been born and what will be born. He stands in front of all beings, whose face is to every side.

5. Before whom there is nothing that is born, who has become all these worlds, the Lord of Creation delighting with creatures, holds to three lights, possessing sixteen forms.

6. By whom Heaven is sublime and the Earth made firm, by whom the Sun-world is upheld and the firmament, who is the measuring force in the region of the atmosphere; to the Unknown God may we give our offering.

7. Whom Heaven and Earth, roaring and standing firm, look up to, trembling in mind, where the Sun rising shines; to the Unknown God may we give our offering.

8. The loving Sun saw in secrecy that mysterious Being, where all the universe becomes a single nest. In him all this converges,

from him all this diverges, who is the warp and weft, the pervasive power in creatures.

9. May the angel, the knower, declare the immortal nature, the being carried diversely in secrecy. Three stations of his are hidden in mystery. He who knows them will become the father of his own father.

10. He is our friend, our father and ordainer, who knows the dominions of all the worlds, where the Gods attaining immortality into the third nature merge.

11. Encompassing all beings, encompassing all worlds, encompassing all the directions of space, in the presence of the first born of truth, by the Self he entered into the Self.

12. Travelling around Heaven and Earth in an instant, around the worlds, the regions of space and the domain of light, having cut the extended chain of karma, he saw That, he became That, he was That.

13. The wonderful lord of being and non-being, the delightful love of the perceiver, may I gain the victorious wisdom, Swaha!

14. Which wisdom Goddess the hosts of the Gods and the ancestors worship. By that Goddess of wisdom, oh sacred Fire, make me full of wisdom, Swaha!

15. May the Lord of the ocean grant me wisdom, may the Fire and the Lord of Creation. May the perceiver and the Spirit grant me wisdom. May the Ordainer grant me wisdom, Swaha!

16. May both the spiritual and ruling orders attain the glory of the Goddess. May the Gods grant that supreme beauty to me. To her, to you, Swaha!

ATHARVA VEDA X.8.

This is part of the second hymn to Skambha, the Divine Pillar or truth of Oneness, from the tenth book of the *Atharva Veda*. Some of these verses were used in the Upanishads or became the basis for Upanishadic teachings.

27. You are the woman and you are the man. You are the boy and you are the girl. You are the old man who totters on his staff. You are born with your face to every side.

28. And you are their father and you are their son. You are the eldest and the youngest. The One God has entered into the mind. Born at first he wakes within the child.

29. From the infinite, the infinite arises. The infinite through the infinite is poured. And may we know that today from which the infinite overflows.

30. She is the eternal, who is perpetually born. She is the ancient one who has encompassed all beings. The great Divine Dawn shining, by the blinking of her eyes envisions all things.

31. Encompassed by the law of truth, as the Divine nature she appears. By her beauty these green trees are garlanded with leaves.

32. That which is near one does not abandon. That which is near one does not see. Perceive the wisdom of the God. He does not die, nor does he grow old.

33. Impelled by that which has nothing before it, the Goddesses declare the Divine Words as they are. As they speak so they attain. That they call the supreme reality.

34. Where Gods and men are lodged like spokes within a wheel, I ask you, where is the flower of the waters, which is hidden by illusion?

35. Impelled by what powers does the wind blow, who holds the five directions together, which Gods look beyond the offering, who are they?

36. The One pervades this earth. The One encompasses the atmosphere, who as the ordainer holds heaven. All directions come together in the One.

37. Who knows the extended thread in whom all these creatures are woven, who knows the thread behind the thread, he knows the supreme reality.

38. I know the extended thread in whom all these creatures are woven. I know the thread behind the thread and that which is the supreme reality.

ISHA UPANISHAD

This is the shortest but one of the most beautiful of the Upanishads in its entirety.

1. All the universe exists as an expansion for the Spirit, whatsoever changing thing there is in this changing world. Experiencing life through that renunciation do not desire what any man has.

2. Doing only sacrificial action here one may wish to live a hundred years. Only thus it is and not otherwise that karma does not cling to a man.

3. Sunless are those worlds, enveloped in blinding darkness, where they go upon departing who are slayers of their own Self.

4. One only, unmoving, swifter than the mind, the senses cannot reach him who moves front. Standing still he speeds beyond all things that run. In him the Lord of life sustains the waters of creation.

5. That moves; that moves not. That is far; that is near. That is within all beings and That is outside all beings.

6. He who sees all beings in the Self and the Self in all beings, henceforth has no more distress.

7. In whom the Self has become all beings, where can there be any delusion, any sorrow, for that man of discernment who sees only the Oneness?

8. He is all-encompassing, luminous, bodiless, without organs, beyond disease, pure and untouched by evil. The Seer, the guide of the mind, all-pervading, self-existent, he ordained all objects according to their nature from eternal equanimity.

9. Into blinding darkness enter those who worship ignorance. Into even greater darkness, as it were, fall those who are attached to knowledge.

10. Ignorance is of one movement, they declare, and knowledge of the other. Thus have we heard from the wise who related to truth to us.

11. The knowledge and the ignorance, who knows them both together, crossing over death through the ignorance, attains immortality through the knowledge.

12. Into blinding darkness enter those who worship destruction. Into even greater darkness, as it were, fall those who are attached to creation.

13. Destruction is of one movement, they declare, and creation of the other. Thus have we heard from the wise who related the truth to us.

14. Creation and destruction, who knows them both together, crossing over death through destruction, attains immortality through creation.

15. The face of truth is covered by a golden vessel. Remove that, oh Sun who nourishes all, that we may perceive our real nature.

16. Sun, our Father, solitary seer, death, who control the power of creation, disperse your rays and gather up your heat that I may see your most beneficent form. The Being in the Sun, He am I!

17. Let my life enter the immortal life and the body end in ashes. Om, Intelligence remember, remember your labor; Intelligence remember, remember your labor.

18. Fire, lead us by the perfect path to reality, God who knows all the ways of wisdom. Remove from us the wandering evil. The most full utterance of surrender may we offer unto you.

Om, Shanti, Shanti, Shanti!

Om, Peace, Peace, Peace!

SANSKRIT
TERMS

Advaita Vedanta	non-dualistic form of Vedantic philosophy
Agamas	Shaivite scriptures
Agni	Vedic sacred fire
Ananda	bliss
Anna	food
Aranyaka	Vedic forest texts
Artha	pursuit of wealth
Aryan	people of spiritual values
Asanas	yogic postures
Ashram	state or stage of life
Atharva Veda	fourth Veda
Atman	the Divine Self
Avatar	incarnation of God
Ayurveda	Vedic medicine
Bhagavad Gita	scripture of the avatar Krishna
Bhakti Yoga	Yoga of Devotion
Bhuktis	planetary time periods, minor
Brahmacharya	control of sexual energy; state of life of learning and purity
Brahma	form of the Hindu trinity governing creation
Brahman	the Absolute or ultimate reality
Brahmanas	Vedic ritualistic texts
Brahmins	people of spiritual values
Brihaspati	Vedic God of the ritual, the planet Jupiter

Buddha	ninth avatar of Vishnu
Buddhism	non-orthodox form of Vedic-Aryan teaching founded by the Buddha or enlightened one
Chakras	nerve centers of the subtle body
Charvakas	materialistic philosophers of ancient India
Cit	consciousness
Dashas	planetary time periods, major
Dharana	yogic concentration or attention
Dharma	teaching or religion; honor or status
Dhatus	bodily tissues in Ayurvedic Medicine
Dhyana	meditation
Doshas	biological humors of Ayurvedic Medicine
Durga	the Goddess as the destroyer of demons
Ganesh	elephant faced God who destroys all obstacles
Gayatri	Vedic chant for awakening the soul
Grihastha	householder stage of life
Gunas	prime qualities of nature
Guru	spiritual teacher
Hanuman	the monkey God
Hatha Yoga	Yoga of the physical body
Hinduism	modern name for the Vedic teaching
Homa	Vedic worship, Fire offerings
Hum	great mantra of Agni and Shiva
Indra	Vedic God of being or life
Ishwara	the cosmic Creator
Itihasas	Hindu epics
Jainism	nonorthodox form of Vedic-Aryan teaching emphasizing non-violence
Jnana Yoga	Yoga of Knowledge
Jyotish	Vedic astrology

Kailas	the world mountain
Kali	the dark form of the Goddess
Kali Yuga	dark or iron age
Kalki	tenth avatar of Vishnu
Kama	pursuit of desire
Kapha	biological water humor
Kapila	great Hindu sage, founder of the Sankhya system of philosophy
Karakas	planetary significators
Karma	Law of Cause and Effect
Karma Yoga	Yoga of Work or Service
Kashmiri Shaivism	Shaivite philosophy of medieval Kashmir
Ketu	south node of the Moon, dragon's tail
Krishna	eighth avatar of Vishnu
Kriya Yoga	yoga of technique
Kshatriya	people of political values
Kundalini	serpent power, power of subtle body
Lakshmi	Goddess of prosperity and beauty; consort of Vishnu
Lalita	Goddess of bliss
Laya Yoga	Yoga of absorption into the sound-current (nada)
Mahabharata	epic story of Krishna
Mahavakyas	great sayings of Vedantic knowledge
Mahayana	great vehicle, northern school of Buddhism
Manas	mind or emotion
Mantra	spiritual or empowered speech
Manu	Vedic original man, founder of human culture
Marmas	sensitive bodily points used in Ayurvedic treatment
Maya	illusion
Mayavada	doctrine that the world is unreal

Meru	the world mountain
Mimamsa	ritualistic form of Vedic philosophy
Moksha	pursuit of liberation
Nada	the sound current of the subtle body
Nadis	nerves of the subtle body
Nataraj	Shiva as lord of the cosmic dance
Nirvana	liberation, the state of peace
Niyamas	yogic observances
Nyaya & Vaisheshika	Hindu philosophies; two of the six systems
Om	the mantra of the Divine
Pancha Karma	five Ayurvedic purification methods
Parashurama	sixth avatar of Vishnu
Parvati	the consort of Shiva
Patanjali	main teacher of classical Yoga system
Pitta	biological fire humor
Prakriti	great Nature, matter
Prana	breath or life-force
Prana yoga	Yoga of the life-force
Pranayama	yogic control of the breath
Pratyahara	yogic control of mind and senses
Puja	Hindu worship, flower offerings
Puranas	Hindu mythological texts
Purusha	pure consciousness, spirit
Radha	consort of Krishna
Rahu	north node of the Moon; dragon's head
Rajas	quality of energy or agitation
Raja Yoga	integral or royal yoga path of Patanjali
Rama	seventh avatar of Vishnu
Ramayana	epic story of Rama

Rasayana	Ayurvedic rejuvenation methods
Rig Veda	oldest Hindu scripture; Veda of chant
Rishis	ancient Vedic seers
Rudra	terrible or wrathful form of Shiva
Sama Veda	Veda of song
Samadhi	absorption, bliss
Sankhya	Vedic philosophy of cosmic principles
Sanskrit	Vedic and mantric language
Sannyasa	stage of life of renunciation and liberation
Santana Dharma	the eternal teaching; traditional name for the Hindu religion
Saraswati	Goddess of speech, learning, knowledge and wisdom
Sat	being
Sattva	quality of truth or light
Sautrantika	Buddhist philosophy of the momentariness of all things
Savitar	Vedic Sun god as the guide of Yoga
Shakti	the power of consciousness and spiritual evolution
Shankara	the great philsopher of non-dualistic Vedanta
Shiva	form of the Hindu trinity governing destruction and transcendence
Shudras	people of sensate values
Shunyavada	Buddhist philosophy that everything is void
Sita	consort of Rama
Skanda	the war God
So'ham	natural mantric sound of the breath
Soma	Vedic Sun God of bliss
Srotas	channel systems used in Ayurvedic medicine
Surya	Vedic Sun God or god of the enlightened mind
Tamas	quality of darkness and inertia

Tantra	medieval yogic and ritualistic Indian texts
Tara	the Goddess in her role as savior
Upanishads	Vedic philosophical texts
Vaishyas	people of commercial values
Vak	Divine Word, the Goddess
Vanaprastha	hermitage stage of life
Varna	Social Value or Class
Vata	biological air humor
Vedas	ancient scriptures of India
Vedanta	Vedic philosophy of Self-knowledge
Vedic Science	integral spiritual science of the Vedas
Vijnana	intelligence
Vijnanavada	Buddhist philosophy that consciousness alone exists
Vishnu	form of the Hindu trinity governing preservation
Yajna	sacrfices, sacred ritual
Yajur Veda	Veda or ritual or sacrifice
Yamas	yogic attitudes
Yantra	geometrical meditation designs
Yoga	techniques of developing and integrating energy
Yoga Sutras	classical text of Patanjali on Yoga
Yogi	practitioner of yoga
Yugas	world-ages

BIBLIOGRAPHY
SUGGESTIONS FOR FURTHER STUDY

BOOKS

This list is suggestive, as there are hundreds of books on these subjects, many quite useful. The following books have many translations and interpretations. They are not only central to the teaching but have often been rendered into clear modern terms.

Ashtavakra. *Ashtavakra Samhita.*
Krishna, Sri. *Bhagavad Gita.*
Patanjali. *Yoga Sutras.*
Tulsidas. *Ramayana.*
Valmiki. *Ramayana.*
Upanishads.
Vyasa. *Mahabharata.*

Vedic

The books below include many classical texts and scriptures. Several versions of them are available, though the translations are often cumbersome. Some have commentaries which can be quite useful.

Aitareya Brahmana.
Atharva Veda.
Rig Veda.
Sama Veda.
Taittiriya Aranyaka.
Yajur Veda.

Classical — General

Agamas.
Badarayana. *Brahma Sutras.*
Buddha. *Saddharma Pundarika (Lotus) Sutra.*
Jaimini. *Jaimini Sutras (Mimamsa).*
Mahanirvana Tantra.
Manu. *Manu Samhita.*
Markandeya Purana.
Narada. *Bhakti Sutras.*
Shiva Purana.

Vishnu Purana.

Classical — Specific
Bhartrihari. *Vakyapadiya* (Sanskrit).
Charaka. *Charaka Samhita* (Ayurveda).
Jataka Parijata (Vedic astrology).
Panini. *Ashtadhyayi* (Sanskrit).
Parasara. *Brihat Parasara Hora Sastra* (Vedic astrology).
Sushruta. *Sushruta Samhita* (Ayurveda).
Vagbhatta. *Ashtanga Hridaya* (Ayurveda).
Varahamihira. *Brihat Jataka* (Vedic astrology).

Modern
M. *The Gospel of Ramakrishna.* New York, NY: Ramakrishna-Vivekananda Center, 1942.
Talks with Sri Ramana Maharshi. Sri Ramanasramam, Tiruvannamalai, India: Sri Ramanasramam, 1955.
Yogananda, Paramahansa. *Autobiography of a Yogi.* Los Angeles, CA: Self-Realization Fellowship, 1946.

By the Author
Frawley, David. *The Astrology of the Seers, A Guide to Vedic (Hindu) Astrology.* Salt Lake City, Utah: Passage Press, 1990.
Frawley, David. *Ayurvedic Healing, a Comprehensive Guide.* Salt Lake City, Utah: Passage Press, 1990.
Frawley, David. *Beyond the Mind.* Delhi, India: Sri Satguru Publications, 1984.
Frawley, David. *The Creative Vision of the Early Upanishads.* India: David Frawley, 1982.
Frawley, David. *Gods, Sages and Kings:Vedic Secrets of Ancient Civilization.* Salt Lake City, Utah: Passage Press, 1991.
Frawley, David. *Hymns From the Rig Veda.* Delhi, India: Motilal Banarsidass, 1986.
Frawley, David, Vasant, Lad. *The Yoga of Herbs, An Ayurvedic Guide to Herbal Medicine.* Santa Fe, New Mexico: Lotus Press, 1986.

PERIODICALS
Hinduism Today. 1819 Second Street, Concord, CA, 94519.
Yoga Internaltional. Rural Route 1, Box 407, Honesdale, PA 18431.
Yoga Journal. P.O. Box 3755, Escondido, CA 92033.

AYURVEDIC CORRESPONDENCE COURSE

We offer a comprehensive correspondence course in Ayurveda based upon the complementary to *Ayurvedic Healing*. It covers all the main aspects of Ayurvedic Medicine and explains Ayurveda as part of the science of Yoga.

Part I. is Introduction, Historical and Spiritual Background, and a comprehensive examination of Ayurvedic Anatomy and Physiology (Doshas, Dhatus, Malas, Srotas, Kalas, and Organs). Part II. is Constitutional Analysis, Mental Nature, the Disease Process, Examination of Disease, Diagnosis (pulse, tongue, and abdomen) and Patient Examination, Yoga and Ayurvedic Psychology. Part III. is Dietary Therapy, Herbal Therapy, Ayurvedic Therapeutic Approaches (including Pancha Karma), Subtle Healing Modalities of Ayurveda and Practical Application of Yoga Psychology.

The course has been approved by well-known Ayurvedic doctors in India. Additional study tapes are available, as well as options for advanced study.

VEDIC ASTROLOGY CORRESPONDENCE COURSE

Vedic astrology, also called Hindu astrology or Jyotish, is the traditional astrology of India, often used along with Ayurveda and Yoga.

This course teaches the fundamentals of Vedic astrology through an explanation of the planets, signs, houses, aspects, harmonic charts, planetary periods and principles of chart interpretation. In addition, it sets forth the astrology of healing based upon the combined use of Ayurveda and Vedic astrology, explaining remedial measures of diet, herbs, gems, colors, mantras, yantras and deities. Spiritual and karmic aspects of astrology are stressed, astrology as a means of self-knowledge and attunement to the cosmic mind.

The course, perhaps the only one of its kind in this regard, presents the system in clear, practical and modern terms and is adapted toward western culture. Options for advanced study are also available.

For Courses send a S.A.S.E. to:

AMERICAN INSTITUTE OF VEDIC STUDIES
P.O. BOX 8357, SANTA FE, NM 87504-8357

BIODATA

Dr. David Frawley is a modern teacher of the comprehensive system of Vedic and Yogic Science, much like the Vedic seers of old. He is acknowledged as an Ayurvedic healer, Vedic astrologer, teacher of Yoga and meditation, and a Sanskrit scholar. Over the past twelve years he has written many books and articles on the different aspects of Vedic knowledge for publication both in the United States and in India.

His Indian books include *Hymns From the Golden Age* (1986), *Beyond the Mind* (1984) and *The Creative Vision of the Early Upanishads* (1982). His articles have appeared in such Indian periodicals as the *Mountain Path, Glory of India, World Union, Sri Aurobindo's Action, the Advent, The Silent Logos,* and *Ananda Varta.*

His American titles include *Ayurvedic Healing, A Comprehensive Guide* (1989), *The Yoga of Herbs* (1986), *From the River of Heaven* (1990) and *The Astrology of the Seers* (1990). He has written for such periodicals as the *Clarion Call, Yoga News (Unity in Yoga), The Eternal Way* and *The Yoga Journal.* He also has a doctor's degree (O.M.D.) in Chinese medicine and is a published *I Ching* scholar both in the United States and China.

Dr. Frawley is the director of the American Institute of Vedic Studies, which aims to provide educational material for a modern restoration of Vedic knowledge, including Ayurveda, Vedic astrology, Vedic studies and Yoga.

His forthcoming books through Passage Press are: *Songs of the Ancient Seers, Selected Hymns from the Rig Veda; The Song of the Sun, The Upanishadic Vision; Beyond the Mind;* and *Himalayan Origins of Civilization Through the Vedas.*

The following are reviews of his various books on Vedic knowledge published in India:

"Frawley is superb when he discusses in what sense the world is a creation of the word. His note on the Mantra is as chiselled as the Vedic Mantra itself." — M.P. Pandit, *The Mountain Path*

"With such spiritual translation and interpretation of the Vedic mantras, he deserves a place amongst the great spiritual commentators of the Veda like Swami Atmananda, Swami Dayananda, Sri Aurobindo and V.S. Agrawal." — Prof. K.D. Shastri; *Haryana Sahitya Academy Journal of Indological Studies*

"The work is an exceptionally admirable attempt to understand the Vedic vision. After Sri Aurobindo, it is perhaps the most original hermeneutical exercise in Vedic studies." — Dr. S.P. Dugy; *Prabuddha Bharata*

"The author discloses an acute sensitivity for the sound and spiritual meaning of the Vedic mantras." — P. Nagaraja Rao; *The Madras Hindu*

GENERAL INDEX

A

Abhinavagupta, 79
absorption, 134
Acorus calamus, 45
acupuncture points, 43
Aditi, 143
Adityas, 142-143
Advaita Vedanta, 112, 120
Agamas, 139, 149
aggregates, 110
Aghora, 123
Agni, 37, 124, 143
Agni Purana, 148
ahamkara, 110
Aim, 81, 126
Aitareya, 145
Aitareya Aranyaka, 148
Aitareya Brahmana, 147
Aitareya Upanishad, 145
ajna chakra, 104
Allium sativa, 45
almonds, 43
aloe, 44
amalaki, 44
American revolution, 63
Amon Re, 125
anahata chakra, 104
Ananda, 101
Angirasas, 142
anjan, 46
Anna, 101
Apas, 143
Aranyakas, 141, 148
Ares, 124
arishta, 46
arjuna, 45
Armenian language, 75
art, 122
artha, 68

Uddalaka Aruni, 145
Aryan dharma, 27, 125
asana, 112, 131, 132, 134
asava, 46
ascendant, 53
ascent, sound of, 81
ashramas, 72
ashtanga, 111
Ashtavakra Samhita, 120
ashwagandha, 45
Ashwins, 142
Asparagus adscendens, 46
Asparagus racemosus, 46
assent, sound of, 81
Assyria, 64
astral, body, 103; and sheaths, 102; plane, 91, 136; world, 51
astrology, 15
Atharva Veda, 144, 145
Atharvan, 145
Atma vichara, 119
Atmakaraka, 57
Atman, 112
Atmayajna, 144
Atri, 142
attention, 134
Sri Aurobindo, 122
Avadhut Gita, 120
avaleha, 46
Avatars, 124, 125, 126
Ayasya, 145
Ayodhya, 125
Ayurveda, 33, 92, 142; active and passive therapies, 35; anatomy and physiology, 40; background of, 36; and Buddhist medicine, 37; and disease, 36; diseases of the head, 36; eight branches, 36; and healing the mind, 36; and herbs, 44; and immortality, 47; and internal medicine, 36; and life-force, 35; and medication, 36; and pediatrics, 36; and psychiatry, 36; and rejuvenation, 36, 47; and Sankhya, 36; and surgery, 36; and Tibetan medicine, 37; and toxicology, 36;

Iron age, 53
Isha Upanishad, 145
Ishwara, 111, 112
Ishwara Krishna, 109
Ishwara-pranidhana, 129
Islam, 99, 122; cultural influences, 29
Itihasas, 148, 150, 151

J

jaggery, 44
Jaimini, 109
Jain, literature, 75; teachings, 108
Jainism, 26, 27, 113
Jamadagni, 142
Janamejaya, 145
japa, 121
jatamansi, 45
Jnana Yoga, 117; goal of, 118
Judaeo-Christian-Islamic tradition, 17
Judaism, 17, 99
Jupiter, 53
Jyotish, 49

K

Kailas, 151
Kaivalya, 92
Kali, 59, 123, 127
Kali Yuga, 53
Kalika Purana, 148
kalka, 46
Kalki, 125, 126
Kalki Purana, 148
kama, 68
Kanwa, 142
Kapha, 37–38; constitutional type, 39; qualities, 38
kapikacchu, 45
Kapila, 109, 110
karakas, 57
karana sharira, 102
karma, 85, 86, 88, 89, 90, 92, 145; and Vedic science, 92
Karma Yoga, 122, 128
Karttikeya, 124
Kashmiri Shaivism, 79, 120

Katha Upanishad, 145
Kaushitaki Brahmana, 147
Kena Upanishad, 120, 145
kicharee, 44
kirtan, 121
Klim, 127
knowledge, 15, 16, 18, 23, 68, 69, 117; definition of, 119; higher and lower, 118; Hindu and Vedic, 18; inner and outer, 21
Koran, 80, 122, 139
Krishna, 36, 109, 110, 121, 124, 125, 141, 146, 148; time of, 145
J. Krishnamurti, 120
Kriya Yoga, 129
kshatriya, 66, 67
Kundalini, 77, 105, 132, 133, 149, 150; Yoga, 131, 132
Kurdish language, 75
Kurma, 124
Kurma Purana, 148
Kuru kings, 145
kvath, 46
Kwan Yin, 128

L

Lakshmi, 59, 123, 127
Lalita, 127
language, Germanic, 17; Greek, 17; Indo-european, 17; Keltic, 17; Latin, 17; and mantra, 22; ordinary, 78; Sanskrit, 17; Slavic, 17; spiritual, 78
Lao Tse, 119
law, moral, 86; natural, 86
Laya Yoga, 133
learning, 79
legend, 20
liberation, 14, 91
life-force, 34; forms of, 38
light, sound of, 81
Linga Purana, 148
linguistics, 15
love, 120

Rig Veda, 37, 75, 78, 108, 110, 116, 140–145, 149–150; date of, 141; ten books of, 142; three social orders, 66
right attitudes, 134
right observation, 134
rishis, 75; the seven, 142
ritual, 85, 92, 108, 121, 144, 147, 149, 150; in India, 50
rock salt, 44
Rome, 14
root chakra, 132
ruby, 58
Rudra, 59, 123, 143
Rudras, 143
Rukmini, 126

S
Sacchidananda, 102
sacred fire, 143
sacred history and cosmology, 151
Sadashiva, 123
Sahasrapadma chakra, 104
Sama Veda, 144, 145
samadhi, 112, 134
samhita, 141
samsara, 91
samyama, 135
Sanat Kumara, 118, 124, 145
Sanatana Dharma, 26, 29, 116, 121
Sankhya, 77, 109, 110, 113, 120; two ultimate principles, 110
Sankhya Karika, 109
Sannyasa, 72
Sanskrit, 17, 75, 140, 141; age of, 75; form of, 76; language of higer mind, 76; language of mantra, 78; scientific language, 76; Vedic and Classical, 83
Sapta Dhatu, See seven tissues, the
Saraswati, 77, 81, 123, 126, 143
Sat, 102
Sat-Tat-Aum, 123
Sati, 123, 127
sattva, 66, 80, 111

Satya Dharma, 27
Sautrantika, 109, 113
Savitar, 82, 117, 124, 143
science, materialistic and spiritual, 20, 22
scientific method, 20
scripture, 20
Scythes, 14
Scythian language, 75
Self, inner, 92, 103; nature of, 102
self-healing, 34
Self-inquiry, 119
Self-knowledge, 91
self-realization, 14, 27, 145
Self-sacrifice, 144
self-study, 129
senses, control of, 134
Serpent Power, 132
sesame seeds, 44
seven seer families, 142
seven tissues, the, 40
Shabda Brahma Mantra Yoga, 78
Shabda Brahman, 80
Shadannana, 124
shadbala, 56
Shaiva Siddhanta, South India, 120
Shakti, 81
Shamanism, Yoga and channeling, 136
Shambhu, 123
Shandilya, 145
Shankara, 109, 110, 120, 123, 146
shankha pushpi, 46
Shankhayana Aranyaka, 148
Shankhya, principles of cosmic existence, 110
Shanmukha, 124
Sharva, 123
Shatapatha Brahmana, 147
shatavari, 46
shilajit, 46
Shiva, 59, 80, 81, 121–124, 127, 149; in *Rig Veda,* 143
Shiva Nataraja, 124
Shiva Purana, 148

180

From the River of Heaven

visualization, 149
Swami Vivekananda, 13, 120
Vrithragna, 125
Vyasa, 109
Vyasa Krishna Dwaipayana, 141

W

waking state, 80, 103
wealth, 68, 69, 70
western astrology, 52; and Vedic
  astrology, 59
western mystical tradition, 103
white musali, 46
winter solstice, 53
Withania somnifera, 45
word as spiritual path, 77
word of God, 140
world, materialistic view of, 50;
  subtle worlds, 50

Y

Yajna, 116
Yajnavalkya, 145
Yajur Veda, 116, 144, 147, 150
yama, 111, 134
yantra, 149, 150
yellow sapphire, 58
Yoga, 13, 14, 27, 35, 92, 93, 97, 107,
  109, 111, 113, 115, 116, 142, 145;
  ancient form of, 117; astrological,
  49; at time of Krishna, 110; and
  Ayurveda, 33; and chakra work,
  103; and detachment, 135; and discrimination, 135; eight limbs of,
  111; experience in, 135; goal of,

135; Hatha, 13, 33; high tech, 137;
  inner and outer aspects, 135;
  integral path, 116; and life, 117;
  Patanjali's definition, 118; path of
  devotion, 116; path of knowledge,
  116; path of service, 116; path of
  technique, 116; power of, 116; as
  practical application of Vedas, 115;
  practice of, 79; and Shamanism and
  channeling, 136; of sound, 77-79;
  of technique, 130
Yoga of Devotion, 103, 120, 122,
  128, 130, 131
Yoga of Knowledge, 103, 117, 119,
  130-133; basic practice of, 119;
  goal of, 118; teachings of, 120
Yoga of service, 128
Yoga of Technique, 103, 130
Yoga psychology, 82
Yoga Shakti, 79, 116
Yoga Sutras, 109, 116, 120, 131, 134
Paramahansa Yogananda, 13, 59, 122
Yogic knowledge, 119
Yogic method, 20
Yogic teaching, secret, 14
yogis, 25
yogurt, 44
yugas, 53
Sri Yukteswar, 59

Z

Zend Avesta, 139
Zoroastrianism, 27, 125, 139, 145;
  and fire worship, 98
Zen, 120